BLUEPRINTS in
NEUROLOGY

Frank W. Drislane, MD
Associate Professor of Neurology
Harvard Medical School
Neurologist, Comprehensive Epilepsy Center
Beth Israel Deaconess Medical Center
Boston, Massachusetts

Juan A. Acosta, MD
Clinical Fellow in Neurology
Harvard Medical School
Fellow in Clinical Neurophysiology
Beth Israel Deaconess Medical Center
Boston, Massachusetts

Michael Benatar, MBChB, D Phil
Clinical Fellow in Neurology
Harvard Medical School
Chief Resident in Neurology
Beth Israel Deaconess Medical Center
Boston, Massachusetts

Bernard Chang, MD
Clinical Fellow in Neurology
Harvard Medical School
Fellow in Clinical Neurophysiology
Beth Israel Deaconess Medical Center
Boston, Massachusetts

John Croom, MD, PhD
Clinical Fellow in Neurology
Harvard Medical School
Chief Resident in Neurology
Beth Israel Deaconess Medical Center
Boston, Massachusetts

Louis R. Caplan, MD
Professor of Neurology
Harvard Medical School
Chief, Cerebrovascular Diseases
Beth Israel Deaconess Medical Center
Boston, Massachusetts

Blackwell
Publishing

© 2002 by Blackwell Science, Inc.
a Blackwell Publishing Company

Editorial Offices:
Commerce Place, 350 Main Street, Malden, Massachusetts 02148, USA
Osney Mead, Oxford OX2 0EL, England
25 John Street, London WC1N 2BS, England
23 Ainslie Place, Edinburgh EH3 6AJ, Scotland
54 University Street, Carlton, Victoria 3053, Australia

Other Editorial Offices:
Blackwell Wissenschafts-Verlag GmbH, Kurfürstendamm 57, 10707 Berlin, Germany
Blackwell Science KK, MG Kodenmacho Building, 7-10 Kodenmacho Nihombashi, Chuo-ku, Tokyo 104, Japan
Iowa State University Press, A Blackwell Science Company, 2121 S. State Avenue, Ames, Iowa 50014-8300, USA

Distributors:

The Americas
Blackwell Publishing
c/o AIDC
P.O. Box 20
50 Winter Sport Lane
Williston, VT 05495-0020
(Telephone orders: 800-216-2522;
fax orders: 802-864-7626)

Australia
Blackwell Science Pty, Ltd.
54 University Street
Carlton, Victoria 3053
(Telephone orders: 03-9347-0300;
fax orders: 03-9349-3016)

Outside The Americas and Australia
Blackwell Science, Ltd.
c/o Marston Book Services, Ltd.
P.O. Box 269
Abingdon
Oxon OX14 4YN
England
(Telephone orders: 44-01235-465500;
fax orders: 44-01235-465555)

Acquisitions: Beverly Copland
Development: Julia Casson
Production: Debra Lally
Typeset by SNP Best-set Typesetter Ltd., Hong Kong
Printed and bound by Capital City Press
Printed in the United States of America

Manufacturing: Lisa Flanagan
Marketing Manager: Kathleen Mulcahy
Cover Design by Hannus Design

02   03   04   05   5   4   3   2   1

The Blackwell Science logo is a trade mark of Blackwell Science Ltd.,
registered at the United Kingdom Trade Marks Registry

Library of Congress Cataloging-in-Publication Data

Blueprints in neurology / by Frank W. Drislane . . . [et al.].
    p. ; cm. – (Blueprints USMLE steps 2 & 3 review series)
   ISBN 0-632-04539-6 (pbk.)
   1. Neurology – Examinations, questions, etc.   2. Physician – Licenses – United States – Examinations – Study guides.
   [DNLM: 1. Nervous System Diseases – Outlines.   2. Neurology – Outlines.   WL 18.2 B658 2002]
  I. Drislane, Frank.   II. Blueprints.
   RC336 .B575 2002
   616.8′0076 – dc21
                                                                    2001007462

RINTS
LOGY

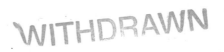

Contents

Preface

Neurology is a wonderful field of study. For over a century it has helped us understand human behavior in all senses, from walking to thinking to illness affecting people most personally, and for several decades it has become an increasingly therapeutic field of medicine. With the aging of the population and the ever increasing value that most people place on the workings of their brains and nervous systems, neurology is likely to assume an ever greater importance in medical education. Nevertheless, it can be complicated, and there can be an intimidating amount of neurology for a new physician to learn. Our purpose in writing this book has been to provide medical students with a reasonably compact review of neurology for practical use while retaining an appreciation for some of the complexity and insights that make the field so fascinating. The authors are all neurologists who have been involved in teaching medical students about neurology, attempting to clarify without oversimplifying. Most of us completed residency recently and are still close enough to examinations at the end of medical school to hope that we remember what is needed and helpful.

Blueprints in Neurology is organized in two major sections. The earlier chapters deal with general principles guiding the neurologic investigation and major neurologic symptoms that bring patients to medical attention. The rest of the book focuses on discrete groups of neurologic illnesses. Board format questions and answers are included to help you review content and prepare for Boards.

We owe plentiful thanks to many people. They include our patients who show us new and complicated symptoms and let us know whether these principles are really true. They include our colleagues and teachers at Beth Israel Deaconess Medical Center and elsewhere. They include Julia Casson and Debra Lally at Blackwell Publishing who did not seem to lose faith that we would complete the volume at some reasonable point. They also include our students who show us how to learn neurology and provide wonderful questions to clarify our own thinking. Finally, we owe major gratitude to our families who volunteered, or at least accepted, our many hours spent on the project.

We hope that you find *Blueprints in Neurology* informative and useful. We welcome feedback and suggestions you may have about this book or any in the *Blueprints* series. Send to *blue@blacksci.com*

Frank W. Drislane, MD
Juan A. Acosta, MD
Michael Benatar, MBChB, D Phil
Bernard S. Chang, MD
John Croom, MD, PhD
Louis R. Caplan, MD

Reviewers

Sean Armin
UCLA School of Medicine
Class of 2003
Los Angeles, California

Ana Burgos, MD
Georgetown University Hospital
Department of Pediatrics
Washington, DC

Kenneth Galeckas, MD
LT, MC, USNR
Medical Officer
Naval Medical Center
Portsmouth, Virginia

Brendan Kelley
Ohio State University
Class of 2002
Columbus, Ohio

Markus Leong, MD
Department of Emergency Medicine
Beth Israel Medical Center
Albert Einstein School of Medicine
New York, New York

Part I
Basics of Neurology

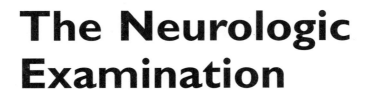

The Neurologic Examination

To practicing neurologists, the neurologic exam reflects the uniqueness of the specialty. In a world of technology, it remains a purely clinical tool still unmatched in its ability to identify and localize abnormalities of the nervous system. To students, however, the exam can be both mystifying and bemusing, an endless series of maneuvers designed to elicit seemingly obscure and inexplicable findings.

When its principles and elements are presented simply, though, the exam is logical and elegant, reflecting the rational diagnostic process that characterizes not just neurology but all of medicine.

PRINCIPLES

1. *The neurologic exam is not a standardized checklist.* Part of the intimidation of performing the exam is its sheer length; hours could be spent on examining the mental status alone. In reality, however, the exam is used in a focused and thoughtful way, depending on what hypotheses have been generated about the patient's disease from the history. A patient presenting with confusion may need quite a comprehensive mental status exam, whereas a patient presenting with a left foot drop may need detailed motor, sensory, and reflex testing of the left leg. In both cases general screening elements of the remaining parts of the exam may be sufficient.

2. *Observation is more important than confrontation.* Most abnormalities of the nervous system manifest themselves in ways visible to the observant examiner. A significant anomia becomes evident when a patient uses circumlocutions to relate his history, and proximal weakness is obvious when he has difficulty arising from a chair. It is often more useful to describe a patient's observed activities and capabilities than to describe the findings obtained upon formal testing. Confrontation testing is subjective and variable; the grading of muscle strength depends on the examiner's effort and expectations of what the patient's "normal" strength should be. The observation of a pronator drift, for example, is less subjective.

3. *The object is to localize.* The extent and complexity of the nervous system require that any attempt to formulate a concise differential diagnosis must begin with an accurate localization of the problem to a specific region of the nervous system. Left hand weakness may stem from carpal tunnel syndrome, a brachial plexus injury, cervical spondylosis, or a right middle cerebral artery stroke, all of which have different diagnostic workups, treatments, and prognoses. The alert physician thinks, What signs would be present in a carpal tunnel problem that would not be present in a brachial plexus problem (and vice versa)? Those signs are then sought, and the exam further refined if necessary.

4. *Not all findings have equal importance.* A common difficulty is that completion of the exam results in a long list of many minor abnormalities of questionable importance, such as a 20% decrease in temperature sensation

over a patch on the left thigh. Although certainly in some cases incidental findings may be the clue to a previously unsuspected diagnosis, in most cases the highest importance must be given to findings directly related to the patient's symptoms and to "hard" findings which require definitive explanation, such as a dropped reflex or a Babinski sign.

◆ KEY POINTS ◆

1. The neurologic exam is not a standardized checklist.
2. Observation is more important than confrontation.
3. The object is to localize.
4. Not all findings have equal importance.

◆ ELEMENTS OF THE EXAM ◆

As discussed earlier, the specific features to include in the neurologic exam should vary with each patient; however, commonly performed elements of the exam are described in this section and listed in Table 1–1.

Mental Status

Neurologists use the mental status exam to identify cognitive deficits that help to localize a problem to a specific region of the brain. Thus the exam differs from that used by psychiatrists, whose objectives in performing the exam are different.

The first step in mental status testing is to assess the level of consciousness. This may vary from the alert wakefulness of a clinic outpatient to the coma of a patient in the intensive care unit. There is a tendency to use "medical" terminology, such as *stuporous*, *obtunded*, or *lethargic*, to describe the level of consciousness, but these have variable meanings; it is more useful to describe how well a patient stayed awake or what stimulation was required to arouse her.

Next, assuming the level of consciousness allows for further testing of cognitive functions, attention is tested, typically with serial forward and backward tasks. These include digit span, reciting the months of the year, or spelling the word *world*, all forward and backward. Attention is usually tested early, because significant inattention

compromises the ability to perform subsequent cognitive tests and may render their interpretation difficult.

Next, language is assessed. As noted previously, listening to the patient tell his history may be all that is necessary to gauge language ability. Formal testing, however, includes assessing the fluency of spontaneous speech, the ability to repeat, the ability to comprehend commands, the ability to name both common and less common objects, and the ability to read and write.

For memory testing, most commonly the patient is given three words and asked to recall them several minutes later, with the aid of hints if necessary. More information can be gained by giving longer lists of words and charting the patient's learning (and forgetting) curve. Visual memory can be tested with three simple shapes for the patient to draw from memory in several minutes.

Visuospatial function can be tested in a variety of ways. Patients can be asked to draw a clock, a cube, or another simple figure; alternatively, they can be asked to copy a complex figure drawn by the examiner (Fig. 1–1).

Neglect is a mental status finding typically not sought by non-neurologists, yet its presence can be a very important sign. Patients with dense neglect may fail to describe items on one side of a picture or of their surroundings, or may fail to bisect a line properly. Subtle neglect may manifest as extinction to double simultaneous stimulation, in which a patient can sense a single stimulus on either side but when bilateral stimuli are presented simultaneously will sense only the one on the non-neglected side.

Tests of frontal lobe function include learning a simple motor sequence of hand postures, inhibiting inappropriate responses when following a "go/no-go" paradigm, or generating lists of words beginning with a particular letter or belonging to a particular category.

◆ KEY POINTS ◆

1. The mental status exam should begin with assessment of level of consciousness and attention, because these can affect the interpretation of subsequent tests.
2. Language, memory, visuospatial function, neglect, and tests of frontal lobe function are other key elements of the mental status exam that can suggest focal brain lesions.

TABLE 1–1

Commonly Performed Elements of the Neurologic Examination

Mental status	
Attention	Serial backward tasks (months of the year, digit span)
Language	Fluency of speech, repetition, comprehension of commands, naming objects, reading, writing
Memory	Three words in 5 minutes
Visuospatial function	Drawing clock, copying complex figure
Neglect	Line bisection, double simultaneous stimulation
Frontal lobe function	Generating word lists, learning a motor sequence
Cranial nerves	
II	Visual acuity, fields, pupils, funduscopic exam
III, IV, VI	Extraocular movements
V, VII	Facial sensation and movement
IX, X, XII	Palate and tongue movement
Motor	
Bulk	Palpation for atrophy
Tone	Evaluation for rigidity, spasticity
Power	Observational tests (pronator drift, arising from chair, walking on heels and toes), direct confrontation strength testing
Reflexes	
Muscle stretch reflexes	Biceps, brachioradialis, triceps, knee, ankle
Babinski sign	Stroking lateral sole of foot
Sensory	
Pinprick and temperature	Pin, cold tuning fork
Vibration and joint position sense	Tuning fork and moving digits
Coordination	
Accuracy of targeting	Finger-to-nose, heel-to-shin
Rhythm of movements	Rapid alternating movements, rhythmic finger or heel tapping
Gait	
Stance	Narrow or wide base
Romberg's sign	Steadiness with feet together and eyes closed
Stride and arm swing	Assessment for shuffling, decreased arm swing
Ataxia	Ability to tandem walk

Cranial Nerves

It is usually easiest to test the cranial nerves (or at least to record the results) in approximate numerical order (Table 1–2).

Olfaction (cranial nerve I) is rarely tested, but when important, each nostril should be tested separately with a non-noxious stimulus, such as coffee or vanilla.

Tests of optic nerve (II) function include visual acuity (using a near card), visual fields (tested by confrontation with wiggling fingers or with a small red object, which is more sensitive), and the pupillary light reflex, the afferent limb of which is mediated by this nerve. Funduscopic examination is the only means by which part of the central nervous system (the retina) can be directly visualized.

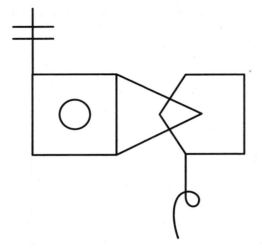

Figure 1–1 Example of complex figure to be copied by patient as test of visuospatial function.

Extraocular movements (III, IV, and VI) are tested by having the patient pursue a moving target that is drawing the letter "H" in front of his face (pursuit), rapidly direct his gaze to various stationary targets (saccades), and fixate on an object while his head is being passively turned (vestibulo-ocular movements). The presence of nystagmus should be noted.

Muscles of mastication (V) are tested by assessing strength of jaw opening and by palpating over the masseters bilaterally while the jaw is clenched. Facial sensation can be tested to all modalities over the forehead (V_1), cheek (V_2), and jaw (V_3). The afferent limb of the corneal reflex is mediated by this nerve.

Muscles of facial expression (VII) are tested by having the patient raise her eyebrows, squeeze her eyes shut, or show her teeth. Though uncommonly tested, taste over the anterior two-thirds of the tongue is mediated by this nerve and can be evaluated with sugar or another non-noxious stimulus.

Hearing (VIII) may be evaluated in each ear simply by whispering or rubbing fingers; more detailed assessment of hearing loss may be accomplished with the Weber or Rinne tuning fork (512 Hz) tests. Vestibular function can be tested in many ways, including evaluation of eye fixation while his head is rapidly turned or by observation for drift in one direction while walking in place with the eyes closed.

Palate elevation should be symmetric and the voice should not be hoarse or nasal (IX and X). Failure of the right palate to elevate implies right glossopharyngeal nerve pathology. The gag reflex is also mediated by these nerves.

Sternocleidomastoid strength is tested by having the patient turn the head against resistance; weakness on turning to the left implies a right accessory nerve (XI) problem. The trapezius muscle is tested by having the patient shrug his shoulders.

Tongue protrusion should be in the midline. If the tongue deviates toward the right, the problem lies with the right hypoglossal nerve (XII).

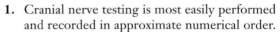

◆ KEY POINTS ◆

1. Cranial nerve testing is most easily performed and recorded in approximate numerical order.

2. Key elements of the cranial nerve exam include assessment of vision and eye movements, facial movement and sensation, and movements of the palate and tongue.

Motor Exam

The motor exam includes more than just strength testing—in fact, strength should usually be the portion of the exam performed last.

First, bulk is assessed by observing and palpating the muscles and comparing both one side to the other and the patient's overall muscle bulk to that expected for age. The presence of fasciculations or of adventitious movements such as tremor or myoclonus should also be noted.

Tone is one of the most important parts of the motor exam. In the upper extremities, tone is checked by moving the patient's arm at the elbow in both flexion-extension and circular movements, by moving the wrist in a circular fashion, and by rapidly pronating and supinating the forearm using a handshake grip. Abnormalities of tone such as spasticity and rigidity are discussed in subsequent chapters. Tone in the lower extremities can be tested well only with the patient supine. The examiner lifts the leg up suddenly under the knee; only in the presence of increased tone will the heel come off the bed.

TABLE 1–2

The Cranial Nerves

Nerve	English Name	Exit Through Skull	Function
I	Olfactory	Cribriform plate	Olfaction (test using non-noxious substance)
II	Optic	Optic canal	Vision (acuity, fields, color), afferent limb of pupillary reflex
III	Oculomotor	Superior orbital fissure	Superior rectus, inferior rectus, medial rectus, inferior oblique, levator palpebrae, efferent limb of pupillary reflex
IV	Trochlear	Superior orbital fissure	Superior oblique (of contralateral eye)
V	Trigeminal	Superior orbital fissure (V_1), foramen rotundum (V_2), foramen ovale (V_3)	Muscles of mastication, tensor tympani, tensor veli palatini, facial sensation, afferent limb of corneal reflex
VI	Abducens	Superior orbital fissure	Lateral rectus
VII	Facial	Internal auditory meatus	Muscles of facial expression, stapedius, taste on anterior two-thirds of tongue, efferent limb of corneal reflex
VIII	Vestibulocochlear	Internal auditory meatus	Hearing, vestibular function
IX	Glossopharyngeal	Jugular foramen	Movement of palate, sensation over palate and pharynx, taste over posterior one-third of tongue, afferent limb of gag reflex
X	Vagus	Jugular foramen	Movement of palate, sensation over pharynx, larynx and epiglottis, efferent limb of gag reflex, parasympathetic function of viscera
XI	Accessory	Jugular foramen	Sternocleidomastoid and trapezius movement
XII	Hypoglossal	Hypoglossal foramen	Tongue movement

Finally, strength or power is assessed, both by functional observation and by direct confrontation (Fig. 1–2). A pronator drift may be observed in an arm held supinated and extended in front of the body. The patient may be asked to rise from a chair without using her arms or to walk on her heels or toes. The power of individual muscles assessed by direct confrontation testing is graded according to the Medical Research Council (MRC) scale (Table 1–3), although refinements of the scale (such as the use of 4–, 4, and 4+) or the use of a ten-point scale increase precision.

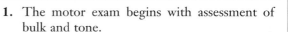

◆ KEY POINTS ◆

1. The motor exam begins with assessment of bulk and tone.
2. Abnormalities of increased tone include both spasticity and rigidity.
3. Strength testing involves both functional observation as well as confrontation testing of individual muscles' power.
4. Strength is graded on the MRC scale from 0 to 5.

MUSCLE POWER TESTING

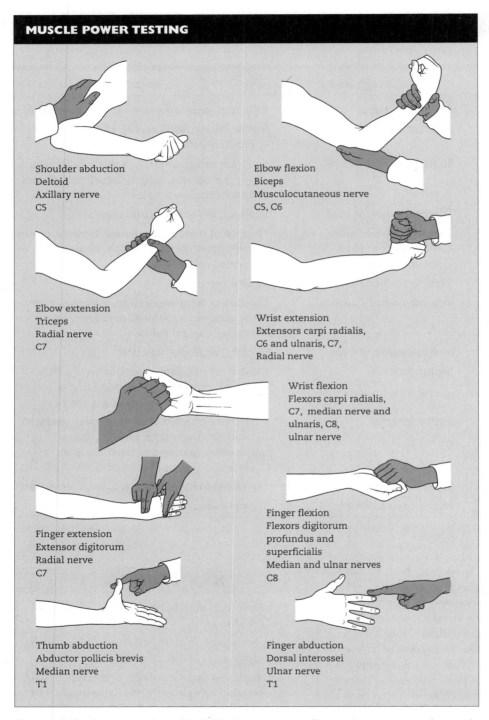

Shoulder abduction
Deltoid
Axillary nerve
C5

Elbow flexion
Biceps
Musculocutaneous nerve
C5, C6

Elbow extension
Triceps
Radial nerve
C7

Wrist extension
Extensors carpi radialis,
C6 and ulnaris, C7,
Radial nerve

Wrist flexion
Flexors carpi radialis,
C7, median nerve and
ulnaris, C8,
ulnar nerve

Finger extension
Extensor digitorum
Radial nerve
C7

Finger flexion
Flexors digitorum
profundus and
superficialis
Median and ulnar nerves
C8

Thumb abduction
Abductor pollicis brevis
Median nerve
T1

Finger abduction
Dorsal interossei
Ulnar nerve
T1

Figure 1–2   Power testing of individual movements. For each movement, the predominant muscle, peripheral nerve, and nerve root are given. (Reproduced with permission from Ginsberg, L. Lecture notes on neurology. 7th ed. Oxford: Blackwell Science, 1999:45–46.)

MUSCLE POWER TESTING (Cont.)

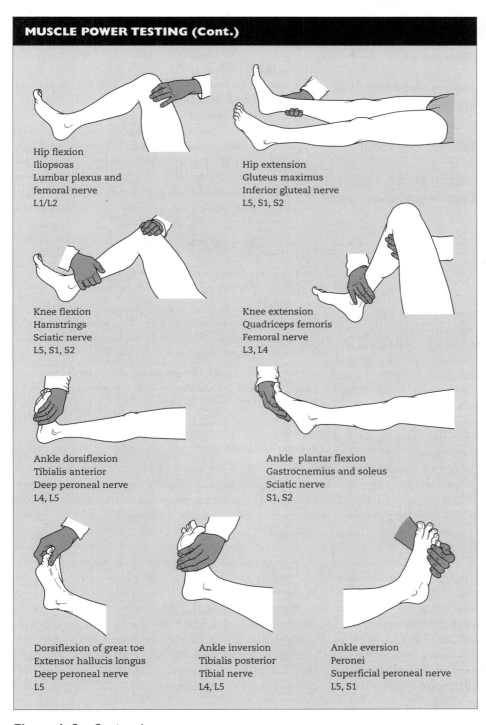

Hip flexion
Iliopsoas
Lumbar plexus and
femoral nerve
L1/L2

Hip extension
Gluteus maximus
Inferior gluteal nerve
L5, S1, S2

Knee flexion
Hamstrings
Sciatic nerve
L5, S1, S2

Knee extension
Quadriceps femoris
Femoral nerve
L3, L4

Ankle dorsiflexion
Tibialis anterior
Deep peroneal nerve
L4, L5

Ankle plantar flexion
Gastrocnemius and soleus
Sciatic nerve
S1, S2

Dorsiflexion of great toe
Extensor hallucis longus
Deep peroneal nerve
L5

Ankle inversion
Tibialis posterior
Tibial nerve
L4, L5

Ankle eversion
Peronei
Superficial peroneal nerve
L5, S1

Figure 1–2   *Continued*

TABLE 1–3

Medical Research Council Grading of Muscle Power

0	No contraction of muscle visible
1	Flicker or trace of contraction visible
2	Active movement at joint, with gravity eliminated
3	Active movement against gravity
4	Active movement against gravity and some resistance
5	Normal power

Reflexes

Muscle stretch (or "deep tendon") reflexes can be useful aids in localizing or diagnosing both central and peripheral nervous system problems (Fig. 1–3).

In the upper extremities, the biceps, brachioradialis, and triceps reflexes are the ones commonly tested. Pectoral and finger flexor reflexes can also be tested. Hoffman's sign is sought by flicking the distal phalanx of the middle finger while observing for flexion of the thumb.

In the lower extremities, patellar (knee jerk) and ankle reflexes are the ones commonly tested. The adductor reflex can also be tested. The Babinski sign is sought by stroking the lateral sole of the foot while observing for extension of the great toe. Clonus, if present, can be elicited by forcibly dorsiflexing the ankle when it is relaxed.

Sensory Exam

The sensory exam can be frustrating to perform because of the tedium of potentially examining the entire body surface (Fig. 1–4), as well as the inherent subjectivity and all-too-frequent inconsistencies in patients' responses.

In general, sensation should be tested in detail in areas relevant to a patient's complaints, especially if the complaints are sensory in nature. Otherwise, screening elements of the sensory exam targeted at the distal lower extremities, where most asymptomatic sensory abnormalities are likely to be found, may be sufficient.

Pinprick sensation is tested with a safety pin, the sharp edge of a broken-off cotton swab, or with special pins designed for the neurologic exam.

Temperature sensation, mediated by the same pathway, is most easily tested with the side of a tuning fork, which if freshly retrieved from an instrument bag will be quite cold on the skin.

Vibration is tested by striking the 128-Hz tuning fork and placing its stem against the joint being tested, typically beginning at the toes.

Joint position sense, or proprioception, is tested beginning most distally by holding the patient's great toe by its sides and moving it slightly upward or downward.

Light touch is the least useful modality to test, because it is carried by a combination of pathways and is unlikely to provide clues to localization or diagnosis.

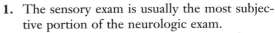

◆ KEY POINTS ◆

1. The sensory exam is usually the most subjective portion of the neurologic exam.
2. In a patient without sensory complaints, screening elements of the sensory exam targeted at the distal extremities may be sufficient.
3. Pinprick and temperature are carried in one pathway; vibration and joint position sense in another.

Coordination

This portion of the exam, often incorrectly referred to as "cerebellar" testing, in fact serves to test coordinated movements whose successful completion requires the interaction of multiple components of the motor system, not just the cerebellum.

Finger-to-nose testing can identify the presence of dysmetria (inaccuracy of targeting) or intention tremor.

Heel-to-shin testing can elicit incoordination in the lower extremities.

Rapid alternating movements, rhythmic finger tapping, or heel tapping are particularly sensitive to coordination problems. Patients may have trouble with the timing or cadence of these movements. *Dysdiadochokinesis* is the term used to describe difficulty with rapid alternating movements.

Gait

Aside from orthopedic surgeons, neurologists are among the only doctors to routinely test a patient's gait, yet the "normal" function of walking requires the proper func-

TENDON REFLEXES

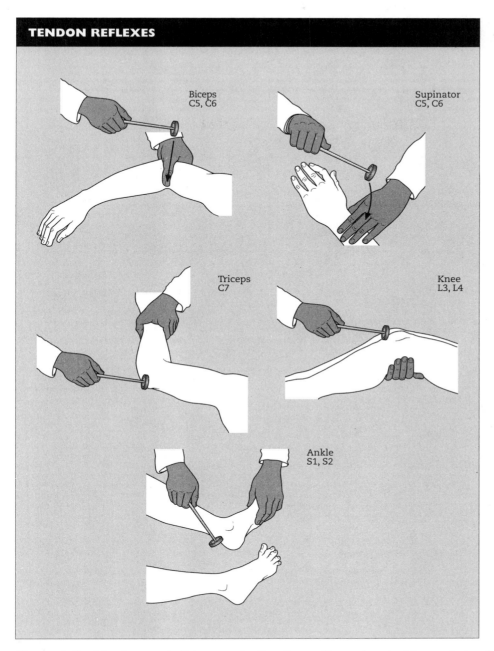

Figure 1–3 Muscle stretch ("deep tendon") reflexes. (Reproduced with permission from Ginsberg, L. Lecture notes on neurology. 7th ed. Oxford: Blackwell Science, 1999:50.)

tioning of so many different aspects of the nervous system that it is frequently a sensitive way to detect an abnormality. In addition, certain diseases such as Parkinson's have quite distinctive gaits associated with them.

The patient with a normal stance maintains the feet at an appropriately narrow distance apart; a wide-based stance is abnormal.

Romberg's sign is present when the patient maintains

DERMATOME DISTRIBUTION

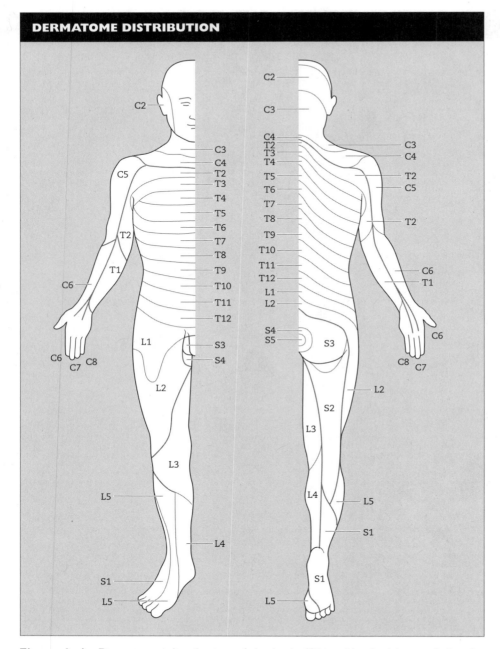

Figure 1–4 Dermatome distribution of the body. (Reproduced with permission from Ginsberg, L. Lecture notes on neurology. 7th ed. Oxford: Blackwell Science, 1999:55.)

a steady stance with feet together and eyes open, but sways and falls with feet together and eyes closed. Its presence usually implies a deficit of joint position sense, not cerebellar function as is commonly believed.

Stride length should be full. Short-stepped or shuffling gaits are characterized by a decrease in stride length and clearance off the ground.

Ataxia of gait results in an inability to walk in a straight line; patients may stagger from one side to the other, or consistently list toward one side. Ataxia is typically associated with a wide-based stance. Ataxia can be brought out most obviously by having the patient attempt tandem gait, walking heel to toe.

The arms normally swing in the opposite direction from their respective legs during ambulation. Decreased arm swing is a feature of extrapyramidal disorders.

Finally, difficulty initiating ambulation or understanding the appropriate motor program for walking, leaving the feet "stuck to the floor" despite intact motor and sensory function, characterizes the gait of frontal lobe dysfunction, sometimes referred to as *gait apraxia*. Hydrocephalus is one etiology of such a gait disorder.

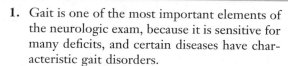

◆ KEY POINTS ◆

1. Gait is one of the most important elements of the neurologic exam, because it is sensitive for many deficits, and certain diseases have characteristic gait disorders.

2. Stance, stride length, arm swing, ability to tandem walk, and initiation of walking should all be assessed in the gait exam.

3. Romberg's sign suggests a deficit in joint position sense.

2 Neurologic Investigations

CEREBROSPINAL FLUID ANALYSIS

Cerebrospinal fluid (CSF) bathes the internal and external surface of the brain and spinal cord. It is produced by the choroid plexus of the ventricles and is absorbed through the villi of the arachnoid granulations that project into the dural venous sinuses. CSF is produced continually at a rate of about 0.5 mL per minute; the total volume is approximately 150 mL. The entire CSF volume is thus replaced about every 5 hours. Lumbar puncture (LP) via the L3-4 interspace is the most commonly used means of obtaining CSF for analysis. LP is contraindicated by the presence of a space-occupying lesion that is causing mass effect or raised intracranial pressure.

Technique

LP is best performed with the patient in the lateral recumbent position with the legs flexed up over the abdomen. Optimal positioning is the key to a successful and atraumatic LP. Ideally, a pillow should be placed between the legs, and the patient should lie on the edge of the bed where there is better support to keep the back straight. The anterior superior iliac spine is at the level of the L3-4 vertebral interspace. The LP may be performed at this level, one interspace higher, or one to two interspaces lower. Remember that the spinal cord ends at the level of L1-2. The needle is inserted with the bevel facing upward so that it will enter parallel to the ligaments and dura that it pierces, rather than transversely cutting them. The needle is directed slightly rostrally to coincide with the downward angulation of the spinous processes. The needle is gently advanced until CSF is obtained. To reliably measure the opening pressure, the legs should be slightly extended and note should be made of fluctuation of the CSF meniscus within the manometer with respiration.

Interpretation of Results

CSF is a clear and colorless fluid. The glucose content is about two-thirds that of blood, and it contains only a trace of protein. Fewer than five cells are present, and these are lymphocytes. Measured by LP in the lateral recumbent position, the opening pressure is about 60 to 150 mm water.

Xanthochromia refers to the yellow discoloration of the supernatant of a spun CSF sample. Its presence helps to distinguish a traumatic tap from *in vivo* intrathecal hemorrhage.

The implications of various CSF findings are summarized in Table 2–1. The CSF findings in a variety of common conditions are summarized in Table 2–2. Special tests may be performed as indicated. Some examples include cytology for suspected malignancy, oligoclonal banding for suspected immune-mediated processes, and a variety of polymerase chain reaction and serological tests for various infectious processes.

TABLE 2–1

Interpretation of CSF Findings

Red blood cells	
No xanthochromia	Traumatic tap
Xanthochromia	Subarachnoid hemorrhage; hemorrhagic encephalitis
White blood cells	
Polymorphs	Bacterial or early viral infection
Lymphocytes	Infection (viral, fungal, mycobacterial); demyelination (MS, ADEM); CNS lymphoma
Elevated protein	Infection; demyelination; tumor (e.g., meningioma); age
Low glucose	Bacterial infection; mycobacterial infection
Oligoclonal bands	Demyelination (MS, ADEM); CNS infections (e.g., Lyme disease); noninfectious inflammatory processes (e.g., SLE)
Positive EBV PCR	Highly suggestive of CNS lymphoma in patients with AIDS or other immunosuppressed states

MS, multiple sclerosis; ADEM, acute disseminated encephalomyelitis; CNS, central nervous system; SLE, systemic lupus erythematosus; EBV PCR, Epstein-Barr virus polymerase chain reaction; AIDS, acquired immunodeficiency syndrome.

TABLE 2–2

CSF Findings in Common Neurologic Diseases

Disease	CSF Findings			
	Pleocytosis	Protein	Glucose	Other
Guillain-Barré syndrome	Absent	↑ (degree depends on the interval from symptom onset)	Normal	—
Viral meningitis, viral encephalitis	Lymphocytes	↑	Normal	Viral PCR
Bacterial meningitis	Polymorphs	↑	Low	—
Multiple sclerosis	Few lymphocytes	Slightly ↑	Normal	OCBs may be present
ADEM	Lymphocytes or polymorphs ↑ (may vary from slight to marked)	Usually ↑ (may be marked)	Normal	OCBs may be present
SAH	Lymphocytes ↑ (reactive to presence of blood)	May be ↑	Normal	Xanthochromia

CSF, cerebrospinal fluid; PCR, polymerase chain reaction; OCB, oligoclonal bands; ADEM, acute disseminated encephalomyelitis; SAH, subarachnoid hemorrhage.

Safety, Tolerability, and Complications

Cerebral or cerebellar herniation may occur when lumbar puncture is performed in the presence of either a supratentorial or infratentorial mass lesion. A computed tomographic (CT) scan should be performed prior to an LP except in cases of suspected meningitis and when a CT scan cannot be performed. Low pressure headache is the most common complication of lumbar puncture and is most effectively treated by having the patient lie flat and increase her intake of liquids and caffeine. Rarely, it may be necessary to administer an epidural blood patch.

◆ KEY POINTS ◆

1. A CT scan should be performed prior to lumbar puncture except when bacterial meningitis is suspected.
2. Lumbar puncture is performed at or below the L2-3 interspace.
3. Xanthochromia indicates recent intrathecal hemorrhage.

COMPUTED TOMOGRAPHY AND MAGNETIC RESONANCE IMAGING

Technical Considerations

Computed tomography is a technique that involves characterization of the degree of x-ray attenuation by tissue. Attenuation is defined simply as the removal (by absorption or scatter) of x-ray photons and is quantified on an arbitrary scale (Hounsfield units) that is represented in shades of gray. Differences in the shades directly reflect the differences in x-ray attenuation of different tissues, a property that depends on their atomic number and physical density. Images are usually obtained in either an axial or coronal plane. Three-dimensional reconstruction and angiography are possible with new-generation spiral CT scanners.

Magnetic resonance imaging (MRI) is similar to CT in that radiant energy is directed at the patient and is detected as it emerges from the patient. MRI differs, however, in its use of radio frequency pulses rather than x-rays. The images in MRI result from the varying intensity of radio wave signals emanating from tissue in which

hydrogen ions have been excited by a radio frequency pulse. A detailed understanding of magnetic resonance physics is not necessary for the interpretation of routinely used MRI sequences. It is sufficient to understand that the patient is placed in a magnet and that a radio frequency (RF) pulse is administered. Signal intensity is measured at a time interval, known as *time to echo* (TE), following RF administration. The RF pulse is administered many times in generating an image; the *time to repetition* (TR) is the time between these RF pulses.

Two basic MRI sequences in common usage are T1- (short TE and TR) and T2- (long TE and long TR) weighted images. Fat is bright on a T1-weighted image, which imparts a brighter signal to the myelin-containing white matter. Water (including CSF) is dark on T1 and bright on T2. Gadolinium is the contrast agent used in MRI, and gadolinium-enhanced images are usually acquired with a T1-weighted sequence.

Other MRI sequences in common usage are fluid-attenuated inversion recovery (FLAIR) and susceptibility- and diffusion-weighted imaging (DWI). FLAIR is a strong T2-weighted image, but one in which the signal from CSF has been inverted and is thus of low rather than high intensity. FLAIR is particularly useful for demonstrating early or subtle T2 signal changes such as accumulation of edema. A susceptibility-weighted sequence is one that is sensitive to the disruptive effect of a substance on the local magnetic field. Examples of substances that exert such a susceptibility effect are calcium, bone, and the blood breakdown products ferritin and hemosiderin. Areas of increased susceptibility appear black on these images.

DWI is a technique that demonstrates cellular toxicity with high sensitivity and is most commonly employed in the diagnosis of acute stroke. Areas of restricted diffusion appear bright on DWI. Figure 2–1 provides examples of T1, T2, FLAIR, and DWI images. Magnetic resonance angiography (MRA) provides a noninvasive means of examining blood flow in the intra- and extracranial vasculature.

Clinical Utility

Head CT is often the initial investigation used in a variety of neurologic disorders, including headache, trauma, seizures, subarachnoid hemorrhage, and stroke. The sensitivity of a CT scan for detecting pathology depends on many factors, including the nature and duration of the underlying disease process. The sensitivity for detecting areas of inflammation, infection, or tumor

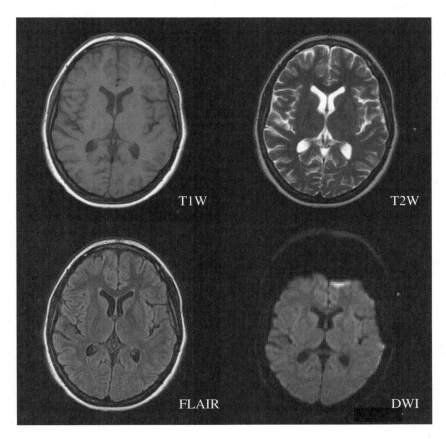

Figure 2–1 Series of MRI scans demonstrating T1- and T2-weighted images, a FLAIR image, and a DWI (diffusion-weighted image).

may be increased by the administration of intravenous contrast. Contrast enhancement indicates local disruption of the blood-brain barrier. CT is the investigation of choice for demonstrating fresh blood.

Apart from providing better anatomic definition, MRI is particularly useful for imaging the contents of the posterior fossa and craniocervical junction, which are poorly seen on CT because of artifact from surrounding bone. DWI is the most sensitive technique available for demonstrating early tissue ischemia and is, therefore, extremely useful in the evaluation of patients with suspected stroke.

Safety, Tolerability, and Complications

CT scanning employs x-rays and is thus relatively contraindicated during pregnancy. The use of RF waves in MRI makes this the imaging modality of choice in pregnant woman. There is no cross-reactivity between the iodinated contrast agents used in CT and the gadolinium used as a contrast agent in MRI. When contrasted

imaging is required, MRI may therefore be preferable when there is a history of allergy to intravenous contrast. Similarly, gadolinium does not have the nephrotoxicity of iodinated contrast. MRI may only be safely used in the absence of metal objects (foreign bodies, plates, and screws) and pacemaker and defibrillator devices. Some people with claustrophobia cannot tolerate MRI; under these circumstances, CT is preferred.

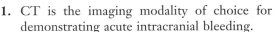

◆ KEY POINTS ◆

1. CT is the imaging modality of choice for demonstrating acute intracranial bleeding.

2. MRI is required for adequate imaging of the posterior fossa and craniocervical junction.

3. DWI is the most sensitive MRI sequence for demonstrating early cerebral ischemia or infarction.

ELECTROENCEPHALOGRAPHY

The electroencephalogram (EEG) provides a record of the electrical activity of the cerebral cortex. Normal EEG patterns are characterized by the frequency and amplitude of the recorded electrical activity, and the patterns of activity correlate with the degree of wakefulness or sleep. The normally observed frequency patterns are divided into four groups: alpha (8–13 Hz), beta (14–30 Hz), theta (4–7 Hz), and delta (0.5–3.0 Hz) (Fig. 2–2). Under normal circumstances, alpha waves are observed over the posterior head regions in the relaxed awake state with the eyes closed. Lower-amplitude beta activity is more prominent over the frontal regions. Theta and delta activity is normal during drowsiness and sleep, and the different stages of sleep are defined by the relative proportions and amplitudes of theta and delta activity.

Technique

The standard EEG is recorded from electrodes attached to the scalp in a symmetrical array. The pattern with which these electrodes are connected to each other is referred to as the *montage*, of which there are essentially two types: bipolar and referential. In a bipolar montage, all electrodes are active and a recording is made of the difference in electrical activity between two adjacent electrodes. In a referential montage, the electrical activity is recorded beneath the active electrode relative to a distant or common average electrode.

Clinical Utility

To appreciate the utility of the EEG, it is important to understand its limitations. First, the patterns of electrical activity recorded by the EEG are rarely (if ever) specific to their cause. For example, the presence of diffuse theta or delta activity during the awake state suggests an encephalopathy, but does not indicate the etiology. Second, the EEG records the electrical activity of cortical neurons. Although subcortical structures influence cortical activity, the surface EEG may be insensitive to dysfunction of deep structures. For example, seizures originating in the medial frontal or temporal lobes may not be readily apparent on the surface EEG. Furthermore, the EEG provides a measure of the electrical activity of the cortex at the time of the recording and is therefore frequently normal in paroxysmal conditions such as seizures. The interictal EEG, for example, may only be abnormal in about 30% of adults with epilepsy. The frequency of interictal EEG abnormalities may be higher in certain forms of epilepsy.

Several common patterns of abnormal activity are recognized. Focal arrhythmic or polymorphic slow activity in the theta or delta range suggests local pathology in the underlying brain. Generalized arrhythmic slow activity indicates diffuse encephalopathy. Interictal epileptiform findings include sharp and spike wave discharges, with or without an accompanying slow wave. Electrographic seizures may take various forms. The most common are rhythmic spike or sharp and slow wave discharges or rhythmic slow waves. These may be focal or generalized.

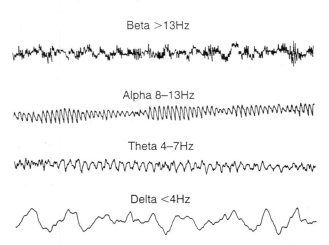

Beta >13Hz

Alpha 8–13Hz

Theta 4–7Hz

Delta <4Hz

Figure 2–2   Electroencephalographic frequencies.

◆   KEY POINTS   ◆

1. Alpha frequency (8–13 Hz) is the dominant posterior rhythm in the awake restful state with the eyes closed.

2. Epilepsy is a clinical diagnosis; interictal EEG findings are only demonstrable in the minority of patients with epilepsy.

NERVE CONDUCTION STUDIES AND ELECTROMYOGRAPHY

Nerve conduction studies (NCS) and electromyography (EMG) are appropriately used as an extension of the clinical examination.

TABLE 2–3

Electromyography in Neurogenic and Myopathic Disorders

	Neurogenic	Myopathic
Insertional activity	↑ (active denervation)	Usually normal ↑ (necrotizing myopathies)
Spontaneous activity	↑ (active denervation)	Usually normal ↑ (necrotizing myopathies)
Volitional motor unit potentials	Large amplitude; polyphasic	Small amplitude; polyphasic
Recruitment	Reduced	Usually normal

TABLE 2–4

Nerve Conduction Studies in Demyelinating and Axonal Neuropathies

	Demyelinating	Axonal
Distal latency	Prolonged	Normal
Conduction velocity	Markedly reduced	Normal; may be slightly reduced
CMAP amplitude	Normal or mildly reduced	Reduced

CMAP, compound muscle action potential.

Technique

In performing NCS, an electrical stimulus is applied over a nerve, and recordings are made from surface skin electrodes. For motor studies, the recording electrodes are placed over the end plate of a muscle innervated by the nerve being stimulated. The nerve is stimulated in at least two locations (distal and proximal), and the distance between the two sites of stimulation is carefully measured. The distal latency, compound muscle action potential (CMAP), and conduction velocity are recorded. The CMAP is a recording of the contraction of the underlying muscle. The distal latency is the time interval between stimulation over the distal portion of the nerve and the initiation of the CMAP. Conduction velocity is calculated by measuring the difference in latency to CMAP initiation between proximal and distal sites of stimulation. For sensory studies, the nerve is stimulated at one site, and the sensory nerve action potential (SNAP) is recorded either at a more proximal site (orthograde study) or at a more distal site (anterograde study). Repetitive nerve stimulation studies are used to demonstrate either decremental or incremental CMAP responses in disorders of the neuromuscular junction.

Electromyography involves the insertion of a needle into individual muscles. Recordings are made of the muscle electrical activity upon insertion (insertional activity), while the muscle is at rest (spontaneous activity), and during contraction (volitional motor unit potentials). With increasing strength of muscle contraction, additional motor units are added cumulatively. This process is known as *motor unit recruitment*; the pattern of recruitment is an important measure during EMG. For routine EMG studies, activity is recorded from a group of muscle fibers simultaneously. Single-fiber EMG is the technique used in the investigation of disorders of the neuromuscular junction.

Clinical Utility

NCS and EMG are used primarily to assist in the localization of pathology within the peripheral nervous system and to more clearly define pathophysiology. For example, in the patient who presents with numbness of the fourth and fifth fingers with weakness of the hand, NCS and EMG may help to differentiate a C8/T1 radiculopathy from a lower brachial plexopathy or an ulnar neuropathy. Similarly, the combination of motor NCS, repetitive nerve stimulation, and EMG may help to localize motor dysfunction (i.e., weakness) to the peripheral nerve, the neuromuscular junction, or the muscle (Table 2–3). In the context of a patient with a polyneuropathy, NCS may help to define the relative degree of motor and sensory involvement and to distinguish primary demyelinating from axonal pathology (Table 2–4).

◆ **KEY POINTS** ◆

1. The goal of NCS and EMG is to localize the pathology within the peripheral nervous system.

2. Repetitive nerve stimulation and single-fiber EMG are useful in the diagnosis of disorders of the neuromuscular junction.

Part II
Common
Neurologic
Symptoms

3

The Approach to Coma and Altered Consciousness

The neurologic evaluation and management of a patient with coma or altered consciousness can be intimidating for the student because such patients are usually critically ill and may require prompt intervention. The fundamental principles behind the evaluation of a neurologic problem, however, should not be discarded. On the contrary, an orderly and hypothesis-based approach may be even more important in a comatose patient than in others, given the need for timely diagnosis and the relative limitations on history and examination.

◆ KEY POINTS ◆

1. Coma is a state of unarousable unresponsiveness.

2. It is important to describe a patient's responses to various degrees of stimulation.

3. The Glasgow Coma Scale, which has prognostic value in head trauma patients, is reproducible and easy to use.

DEFINITION

Coma is defined as a state of unarousable unresponsiveness. Typically the patient lies with eyes closed and does not open them even to vigorous stimulation, such as sternal rub, nasal tickle, or nailbed pressure. Alterations in consciousness short of coma are often described using terms such as *drowsiness*, *lethargy*, *obtundation*, and *stupor*, but these terms tend to be used imprecisely and it is generally best to simply describe how the patient responded to various degrees of stimulation. The Glasgow Coma Scale assigns a numerical score to a patient's level of responsiveness and is commonly used by neurosurgeons in cases of head trauma (see Table 17–1 in the chapter on head Injury). Its utility lies in its ease of use by nurses and paramedics, its interrater reproducibility, and its prognostic value following head injury.

CLINICAL APPROACH

An algorithm for approaching patients with coma or altered consciousness is presented in Figure 3–1. The initial steps of stabilization and evaluation culminate in the neurologic exam, which is performed with two goals in mind: to assess brainstem function and to look for focal signs. The differential diagnosis and further investigations stem from this clinical assessment.

1. *Remember the ABCs.* In any patient with altered consciousness, the airway, breathing, and circulation should be checked and maintained according to usual protocols, including intubation and mechanical ventilation if required.

2. *Look for obvious clues to etiology.* A brief history and general exam should be performed to search for obvious clues. A history of medical problems such as diabetes,

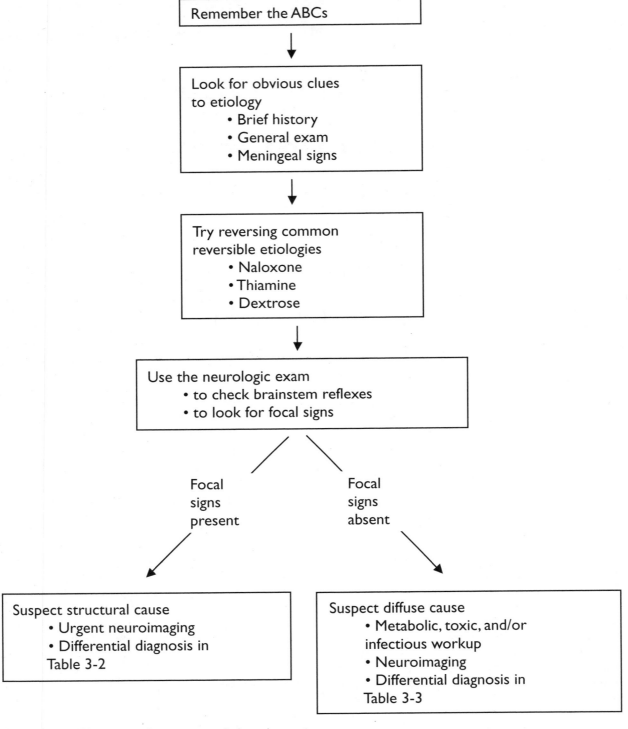

Figure 3–1 The approach to coma and altered consciousness.

hepatic failure, alcoholism, or a seizure disorder may be provided by the family, noted on a medical alert bracelet, or deduced from prescription labels. The circumstances in which the patient was found can offer clues to the onset or etiology of depressed consciousness. The general exam may yield telling signs, such as an odor on the breath, needle tracks on the skin, or a tongue laceration. It is important in any unconscious patient to check for meningeal signs, because both bacterial meningitis and subarachnoid hemorrhage may lead to depressed consciousness.

3. *Try reversing common reversible etiologies.* Most emergency rooms make it standard practice to administer naloxone, thiamine, and dextrose to any patient with depressed consciousness and no obvious etiology. Note that thiamine should always be given before glucose because the latter can precipitate Wernicke's encephalopathy.

4. *Check brainstem reflexes and look for focal signs.* These are the two primary goals of the neurologic exam in this setting, since the subsequent diagnostic and therapeutic steps will depend on these clinical findings.

◆ KEY POINTS ◆

1. The clinical approach to the patient with altered consciousness begins with the ABCs: airway, breathing, and circulation.

2. Look for obvious clues to etiology.

3. Try reversing common reversible etiologies.

4. Use the neurologic exam to check brainstem reflexes and look for focal signs.

EXAMINATION

It is important to proceed with the neurologic exam of a comatose patient in an orderly fashion—it is easy to be intimidated or distracted by the array of attached tubes and lines or by the intensity and anxiety of other clinicians. An appropriate way to begin is to progress systematically through the sequence of the usual neurologic exam, making adjustments as necessary for the patient's altered level of responsiveness.

Mental status testing in these patients begins with assessing the level of consciousness. An increasing gradient of stimulation should be applied and the patient's responses recorded. For example, does he lie with his eyes closed but open them slowly when spoken to in a loud voice? Does he groan but not open his eyes when sternal rub is applied? For many patients, further cognitive testing may not be possible. For those who can be aroused even briefly, however, a short evaluation of attention, language, visuospatial function, and neglect is in order, because this may reveal a gross focal finding such as an aphasia or dense neglect of the left side.

Cranial nerves should be examined in detail, since this is the portion of the exam most relevant to the assessment of brainstem function. In an arousable patient, most cranial nerves can be tested in the usual manner. In a patient who is not arousable enough to follow commands, several important brainstem reflexes should be tested (Table 3–1), including the pupillary, corneal, oculocephalic, and gag reflexes. In addition, funduscopic examination should always be performed. For many patients with altered consciousness, testing for a blink to visual threat may be the only way to judge visual fields. If the patient cannot move the face to command, then the examiner may be restricted to looking for an asymmetry at rest, such as a flattened nasolabial fold on one side. The presence of an endotracheal tube may make such observation difficult, however.

Motor tone should be checked in all extremities. If the patient can cooperate with some testing, a gross hemiparesis can be ruled out by having the patient hold her arms extended or legs elevated, and observing for downward drift. Otherwise, the examiner may be restricted to observing for asymmetry of spontaneous movements (or to ask caretakers if all extremities have been seen to move equally). Failing that, noxious stimuli such as nailbed pressure can be applied to each limb and the speed and strength of withdrawal noted, although abnormalities here may result from sensory loss as well as motor dysfunction. Decorticate and decerebrate posturing, signs of brainstem dysfunction, may be seen either spontaneously or in response to noxious stimuli (Fig. 3–2).

Muscle stretch reflexes can be tested in the usual manner, and Babinski sign should be sought.

Sensory testing in most patients with altered consciousness is limited to testing of light touch or pain sensation. The application of nailbed pressure to each limb, as described previously, may be useful in looking for gross sensory abnormalities.

TABLE 3–1

Brainstem Reflexes

Reflex	Cranial Nerves Involved	How to Test
Pupillary	II (afferent); III (efferent)	Shine light in each pupil and observe for direct (same side) and consensual (contralateral side) constriction
Oculocephalic (doll's eyes)	VIII (afferent); III, IV, VI (efferent)	Forcibly turn head horizontally and vertically and observe for conjugate eye movement in opposite direction (contraindicated if cervical spine injury has not been ruled out)
Caloric testing (if necessary)*	Same	Inject 50 mL ice water into each ear and observe for conjugate eye deviation toward the ear injected
Corneal	V I (afferent); VII (efferent)	Touch lateral cornea with cotton tip and observe for direct and consensual blink
Gag	IX (afferent); X/XI (efferent)	Stimulate posterior pharynx with cotton tip and observe for gag

*Caloric testing should be performed if turning the head is contraindicated or does not result in eye movement. Never assume the eyes are immobile unless caloric testing has been done.

Coordination and gait may be tested in patients who are arousable enough.

◆ KEY POINTS ◆

1. The mental status exam in patients with altered consciousness primarily assesses the level of responsiveness.
2. The cranial nerve exam includes the testing of important brainstem reflexes, including the pupillary, corneal, and oculocephalic reflexes.
3. The remainder of the examination should be dedicated to looking for focal abnormalities.

DIFFERENTIAL DIAGNOSIS

There are two main ways in theory in which consciousness can be depressed: The brainstem can be dysfunctional, or both cerebral hemispheres can be dysfunctional simultaneously. And, in fact, acute pathology in the brainstem (e.g., pontine hemorrhage) can lead to coma, as can processes affecting both cerebral hemispheres at once (e.g., hypoglycemia). However, unilateral cerebral hemisphere lesions, if large or severe enough to cause swelling and compression of the opposite hemisphere or downward pressure on the brainstem, can also lead to coma.

Therefore, most neurologists interpret the information obtained from the exam of the comatose patient using the following principle: The presence or absence of brainstem reflexes suggests how deep the coma is, while the presence or absence of focal signs narrows the differential diagnosis and guides the workup.

Thus, in milder cases of depressed consciousness, the pupillary, corneal, and gag reflexes may all be preserved. In more severe cases, some or all of these brainstem reflexes may be lost, no matter what the etiology. (Note that if a brainstem reflex is abnormal in an asymmetric fashion, such as a unilateral unreactive pupil, this would

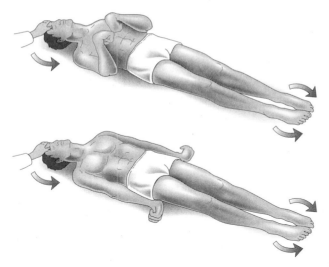

Figure 3–2   Decorticate (above) and decerebrate (below) posturing in response to noxious stimuli. Both indicate brainstem dysfunction, although decorticate posturing suggests dysfunction slightly more superior than decerebrate posturing. (Reproduced with permission from Kandel ER, Schwartz JH, Jessell TM. Principles of neural science. 4th ed. New York: McGraw-Hill, 2000:903.)

be interpreted as a focal sign and suggests compression of or primary pathology in the brainstem.)

The presence of focal signs on either cranial nerve testing or the remainder of the examination, including such findings as hemiparesis, aphasia, reflex asymmetry, facial droop, or a unilateral Babinski sign, suggests a structural cause of depressed consciousness (Table 3–2). Examples include a large unilateral stroke or intracranial hemorrhage. The absence of focal signs suggests a diffuse cause of depressed consciousness, including metabolic, toxic, or hypoxic-ischemic etiologies (Table 3–3). Examples include coma from fulminant hepatic failure, barbiturate overdose, or anoxia following prolonged cardiac arrest.

◆   KEY POINTS   ◆

1. In theory, consciousness can be depressed either by dysfunction of the brainstem or

---

TABLE 3–2

Structural Causes of Depressed Consciousness

Acute ischemic stroke
  Brainstem
  Unilateral cerebral hemisphere (with edema)

Acute intracranial hemorrhage
  Intraparenchymal
  Subdural
  Epidural

Brain tumor (with edema or hemorrhage)
  Primary
  Metastatic

Brain abscess

---

dysfunction of both cerebral hemispheres simultaneously; in reality, large unilateral hemisphere lesions qualify as well.

2. The presence or absence of brainstem reflexes suggests how deep the coma is.

3. The presence of focal signs suggests a structural cause of coma.

4. The absence of focal signs suggests a diffuse cause of coma, such as metabolic, toxic, or hypoxic-ischemic etiologies.

LABORATORY AND RADIOGRAPHIC STUDIES

The distinction between structural and diffuse causes of depressed consciousness, arrived at by interpreting the findings on exam, suggests different pathways of diagnostic workup.

The presence of focal findings on examination, suggesting a structural cause, demands urgent head imaging, almost always a noncontrast head computed tomographic (CT) scan. One should be looking for signs of a large acute stroke, an intracranial hemorrhage, or a mass lesion that may have rapidly enlarged or had hemorrhage within it. (Contrast-enhanced CT should be avoided if acute blood is possible.) Even in cases in

---

TABLE 3–3

Diffuse Causes of Depressed Consciousness

Metabolic
  Electrolyte abnormality
      Hyponatremia, hypernatremia,
        hypocalcemia, hypercalcemia,
        hypomagnesemia, hypermagnesemia,
        hypophosphatemia
  Glucose abnormality
      Hypoglycemia, nonketotic hyperosmolar coma,
        diabetic ketoacidosis
  Hepatic failure
  Uremia
  Thyroid dysfunction
      Myxedema coma, thyrotoxicosis
  Adrenal insufficiency
Toxic
  Alcohol
  Sedatives
  Narcotics
  Psychotropic drugs
  Other exogenous toxins (carbon monoxide, heavy
    metals)
Infectious
  Meningitis (bacterial, viral, fungal)
  Diffuse encephalitis
Hypoxic-ischemic
  Respiratory failure
  Cardiac arrest
Other
  Subarachnoid hemorrhage
  Carcinomatous meningitis
  Seizures or postictal state

---

which focal brainstem signs are found, the initial choice of head imaging may need to be a CT scan rather than magnetic resonance imaging (MRI), despite the poor quality of the former in evaluating the brainstem, because of the possibility of a large cerebral hemisphere lesion compressing the brainstem and the more rapid availability of CT.

The absence of focal findings on examination, suggesting a diffuse cause, warrants an extensive workup for causes of metabolic, toxic, or infectious etiologies.

Blood testing including complete blood count (CBC), electrolytes, glucose, liver function tests, and toxicologic screen may be necessary. If infection is suspected, a chest x-ray, urinalysis, and blood or urine cultures may be called for. There should be a low threshold for obtaining a lumbar puncture (LP). If a basic workup is unrevealing, one should search for more unusual causes (such as for myxedema coma by checking thyroid function tests). Head imaging is usually needed even in these cases of suspected diffuse cause, because it may demonstrate signs of global hypoxic-ischemic injury, diffuse cerebral edema, or bilateral lesions mimicking a diffuse process, although the urgency is not as high as for patients with focal findings. Of course, a head CT should be performed before obtaining an LP almost without exception in the evaluation of a patient with depressed consciousness, given the risk of precipitating brain herniation if a large intracranial mass, particularly in the posterior fossa, is present. (If bacterial meningitis is suspected, empiric antibiotic treatment can be started if CT scanning may be delayed.)

An electroencephalogram (EEG) is frequently ordered in patients with coma or altered consciousness. Although many of its findings may be nonspecific, the EEG can be of use in helping to assess how deep a coma is, based on the degree of background slowing. In addition, there are occasionally more specific patterns on EEG that suggest a particular diagnosis, such as hepatic encephalopathy or anoxic brain injury. Finally, the EEG can rule out nonconvulsive status epilepticus as a cause of coma in cases in which this is clinically suspected.

◆   KEY POINTS   ◆

1. If a structural cause is suspected, urgent head imaging, usually with noncontrast head CT, should be performed.

2. If a diffuse cause is suspected, an extensive workup for metabolic, toxic, or infectious causes should be undertaken.

3. Head imaging in suspected diffuse cases may demonstrate cerebral edema, signs of global hypoxic-ischemic injury, or bilateral lesions mimicking a diffuse process.

4. Head CT should be performed before LP almost without exception.

5. EEG can assess the depth of coma and can occasionally suggest a specific diagnosis.

2. The lowering of intracranial pressure may be a neurologic emergency if the patient shows signs of brain herniation.

3. Prognostic factors for coma or altered consciousness include both etiology and patient age.

TREATMENT AND PROGNOSIS

Needless to say, the treatment of coma and altered consciousness rests on the specific diagnosis. Metabolic, infectious, or toxic etiologies require mostly medical management, while some etiologies of structural coma may require neurosurgical intervention. Specific treatments for particular conditions are detailed in later chapters, in particular Chapter 14 for strokes and hemorrhages, Chapter 17 for head trauma, Chapter 18 for systemic and metabolic disorders, Chapter 19 for brain tumors, and Chapter 21 for central nervous system infections.

When increased intracranial pressure (ICP) is suspected clinically or radiographically, treatments aimed at lowering ICP should be applied. These include raising the head of the bed, hyperventilation, and the use of osmotic diuretics such as mannitol. Corticosteroids tend to be useful only in cases of edema associated with brain tumors. The lowering of ICP may be a neurologic or neurosurgical emergency if the patient shows signs of brain herniation, which is discussed in more detail in Chapter 17.

The prognosis of depressed consciousness is mostly dependent on etiology—the patient with a barbiturate overdose may recover completely, whereas one with a severe anoxic injury will likely not. Age is an important prognostic factor as well. One of the most frequent reasons for ICU neurologic consultation is to estimate the prognosis of a patient in coma following cardiopulmonary arrest—in these cases the circumstances and duration of the arrest are important, and published studies have correlated outcome with findings on neurologic examination performed at least 24 hours after the arrest.

◆ KEY POINTS ◆

1. The treatment of coma or altered consciousness depends on etiology.

SPECIAL TOPICS

Persistent Vegetative State

Persistent vegetative state refers to a state in which patients have lost all awareness and cognitive function but may remain with their eyes open, exhibit sleep-wake cycles, and maintain respiration and other autonomic functions. Patients may progress into this state after being in coma for a prolonged period if their vital functions have been supported.

Locked-in Syndrome

Although locked-in syndrome can be confused with coma at first glance, a patient with locked-in syndrome is completely awake and may be cognitively intact with no abnormality of consciousness. Usually a consequence of large lesions in the base of the pons, locked-in syndrome leaves patients unable to move their extremities and most of their face. Patients may be limited to communicating by vertical eye movements or blinks, if all other motor function is lost.

Brain Death

Death can be declared either when there has been irreversible cessation of cardiopulmonary function or when there has been irreversible cessation of all functions of the entire brain, including the brainstem. A declaration of death based on the latter criterion is commonly referred to as *brain death*. Many institutions have specific guidelines for how brain death must be determined, but in general the patient must be comatose, have absent brainstem reflexes, and have no spontaneous respirations even when the Pco_2 has been allowed to rise (the apnea test). Confounding factors such as hypothermia or drug overdose must not be present. Confirmatory tests most commonly include an EEG, which can demonstrate electrocerebral silence ("flat line"), or cerebral angiography, which can demonstrate absence of blood flow to the brain.

◆ KEY POINTS ◆

1. A persistent vegetative state may follow prolonged coma and is characterized by preserved sleep-wake cycles and maintenance of autonomic functions with absence of awareness and cognition.

2. Locked-in syndrome, in which awareness and cognitive function are preserved but almost complete paralysis occurs, is caused by large lesions in the base of the pons.

3. Brain death is a declaration of death based on irreversible cessation of all brain functions.

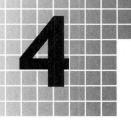

Neuro-Ophthalmology

An understanding of visual impairment, pupillary disturbances, and oculomotor control is essential in the diagnosis of neurologic disorders. Our perception of the outer world requires more than the simple processing of visual information. Visual information is integrated with somatosensory, motor, and auditory information for a maximal interpretation of our environment.

The examination of vision consists not only of evaluating how we see and how we move our eyes, but also of testing the complex integration and analysis of that information. Much of brain function involves looking and seeing. A systematic approach to evaluating patients with "visual" problems includes the analysis of three major processes: vision, oculomotor movements, and integration of visual information. In this chapter we will study the first two; the third constitutes part of higher cortical function discussed elsewhere.

ANATOMY

Visual perception begins in the retina after the light enters the cornea. Light stimulates the rods and cones in the retina, where the visual stimuli are converted into electrical signals that are sent through the optic nerve to centers in the brain for further processing. The visual pathway is shown in Figure 4–1.

The human brain is dominated by visual function, and the brain is organized accordingly. The more posterior part of the cerebral hemispheres is in charge of seeing and analyzing visual information, including written language, and the more anterior part is in charge of looking at and exploring visual space.

Ninety percent of retinal axons terminate in a retinotopic fashion in the lateral geniculate nucleus, the principal subcortical structure that carries visual information to the cerebral cortex through the optic radiations. The primary visual cortex is visual area 1 (V1), corresponding to Brodmann's area 17 or striate cortex. It receives information exclusively from the contralateral visual hemifield. This produces a coherent visual image. The information is then transferred to associative visual cortex, including areas 18 and 19, and to many higher-order centers in the posterior parietal and inferior temporal cortices. Here the perception of motion, depth, color, location, and form takes place.

Understanding gaze control includes not only eye movements but also other neuronal control systems that keep the fovea on target. It is necessary to know the six muscles that move the eyes, and also the elements involved in fixation, saccades, smooth pursuit, and vergence.

SYMPTOMS APPROACH TO NEURO-OPHTHALMOLOGIC DISTURBANCES

The most common neuro-ophthalmologic symptoms are loss of vision and diplopia. The nature of these symptoms should be clarified in order to localize the

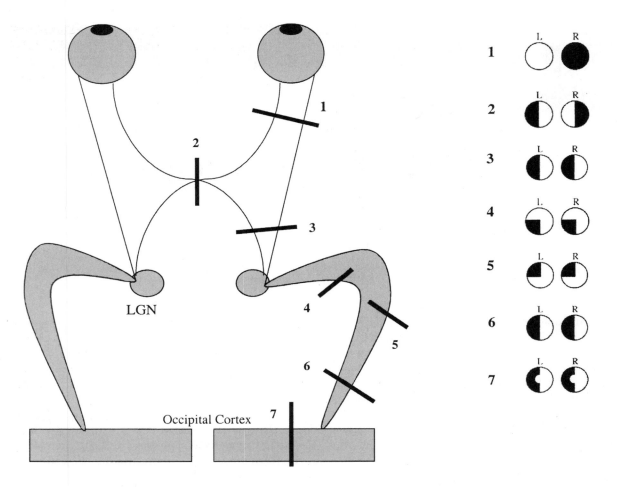

Localization	Visual field defect
1. Optic nerve	1. Right eye blindness
2. Chiasm	2. Bitemporal visual field defect
3. Optic tract	3. Left homonymous hemianopia
4. Optic radiations (parietal)	4. Left inferior homonymous quadrantonopia
5. Optic radiations (temporal or Meyer's loop)	5. Left superior homonymous quadrantonopia
6. Optic radiations (both)	6. Left homonymous hemianopia
7. Occipital cortex	7. Left homonymous hemianopia with macular sparing

Figure 4–1 The visual pathway.

dysfunction. Other symptoms include eye pain, visual hallucinations, and oscillopsia. Two important signs discussed in this chapter are the abnormal optic disc and anisocoria (unequal pupils).

Visual Loss

Visual disturbances can be described as positive or negative phenomena. Positive visual phenomena include brightness, shimmering, sparkling, hallucinations, shining, flickering, or colors, often suggesting migraine or seizures. Negative visual phenomena can be described as blackness, grayness, dim vision, and shade-obscuring vision, as seen in patients with strokes or transient ischemic attacks (TIAs).

When the complaint is loss of vision, the following questions will help to localize the site of pathology.

1. Is this a monocular or binocular problem? Ask the patient if the problem goes away when one eye is closed.
2. Does it affect a portion or the entire visual field?
3. Is it transient or persistent?
4. Were there other associated symptoms, such as headache, visual auras, motor or sensory disturbances, changes in mentation, seizures, or eye pain (e.g., with optic neuritis)?

Clinical Evaluation of Visual Loss

The evaluation of acquired visual loss (Table 4–1) begins with determining whether the problem is at the level of the eye, optic nerve, chiasm, optic tract, lateral geniculate nuclei (LGN), optic radiation, or occipital cortex. Once the site of dysfunction is determined, the workup is targeted to the specific cause.

The diagnostic evaluation includes visual acuity, assessment of color vision, test for afferent pupillary defects, testing of visual fields, and ophthalmoscopic evaluation. The ophthalmoscopic evaluation looks for retinal nerve fiber layer damage, optic atrophy, swollen disc, abnormal optic disc (hypoplastic, tilted, etc.), vascular lesions, and retinal emboli.

To test visual acuity (VA), use a distance chart with good illumination. At the bedside the near chart (handheld Snellen chart) is often enough. If the VA is poor, try using a pinhole (you can create one by perforating small holes in a blank card). If the pinhole test improves the VA, the problem is in refraction. If the patient is unable to read letters, try counting fingers, followed by

---

TABLE 4–1

Causes of Visual Loss

Retina
  Detachment
  Infectious: CMV, toxoplasmosis
  Toxic: ethambutol
  Degenerative: macular degeneration, retinitis
    pigmentosa
  Ischemic: embolic

Optic disc
  AION: vasculitic and nonvasculitic
  Optic neuritis
  Glaucoma
  Papilledema (late)
  Sarcoidosis
  Tumor

Optic nerve
  Demyelination
  Tumor, including meningioma, glioma, etc.
  Thyroid ophthalmopathy
  Trauma

Chiasm
  Tumor: pituitary tumors such as adenoma,
    craniopharyngioma, and glioma
  Sphenoid mucocele
  Internal carotid artery aneurysm
  Trauma
  Demyelination
  Vascular
  Toxic

Retrochiasmal
  Tumor: glioma, meningioma, metastasis
  Stroke involving the visual pathway
  Demyelination
  Degenerative diseases

CMV, cytomegalovirus; AION, anterior ischemic optic neuropathy.

---

perception of movement and finally perception of a bright light. Report the results in that order. Impairment of VA is usually a problem in the refractive apparatus of the eye or the optic nerve, or both. Rarely, chiasmal or retrochiasmal lesions cause changes in VA.

Color vision is tested by using Ishihara plates. Red desaturation (decreased perception of red color) can be seen early in optic nerve problems (particularly optic neuritis).

When testing pupils, report the size of the pupil and its reaction to light, both consensually and in accommodation. Use a bright light. Look for a relative afferent pupillary defect (RAPD).

Visual field testing at the bedside is done by confrontation. Cover one eye at a time. Move your fingers or a small white or red object over the different quadrants and compare the patient's visual field to yours. Match the patient's blind spot against your own using the small white or red pin.

Table 4–2 compares the clinical characteristics of visual loss according to localization.

◆ KEY POINTS ◆

1. Organize your exam when examining vision. Remember to use bright light.

2. Examine one eye at a time.

3. Monocular visual loss implies problems in the eye, optic nerve, or chiasm. Binocular visual loss implies a chiasmal or retrochiasmal lesion.

4. The pattern of visual field loss helps in the localization of the site of the lesion (see Fig. 4–1).

Disorders of the Pupil

Unequal pupil size (anisocoria) is a common finding. If the iris is healthy, the next step will be to distinguish a physiologic from a pathologic anisocoria.

Anatomy

Light activates retinal ganglion cells that send their axons through the optic nerve, chiasm, and optic tract to synapse in the pretectal midbrain nuclei, also known as *Edinger-Westphal nuclei* (EWN) (rostral portion of the third nerve). Efferent parasympathetic fibers from the EWN travel with the third cranial nerve. In the cavernous sinus, they run with the inferior division of the third nerve and ultimately synapse in the ciliary ganglion. The iris contains two muscles that regulate pupil size. The sphincter is a pupilloconstrictor innervated by parasympathetic fibers of the third nerve. The dilator (pupillodilator) is innervated by the cervical sympathetic system. The sympathetic system starts in the ipsilateral posterolateral hypothalamus (first-order neuron) and projects down the brainstem to the intermediolateral cell column at C8-T1 spinal levels. The second-order neurons synapse in the superior cervical ganglion (SCG). Third-order neurons travel along the internal carotid artery into the cavernous sinus and from there into the orbit to the pupillodilator muscles.

Clinical Assessment

Document pupil reactivity and size in bright and dim illumination. Remember that up to 25% of normal people have asymmetric pupils without pathologic significance. In physiologic anisocoria, the amount of anisocoria does not change with different illumination. Pupils should respond normally to light and near stimulation. If the anisocoria is not physiologic, the next question to ask is which pupil is abnormal, the dilated or the constricted one?

First, examine the pupils in the dark (turn the lights off and look at the pupils during the first 5 to 10 seconds). A dilation lag in the small pupil, and anisocoria greater in darkness, means a sympathetic defect in that pupil. Horner's syndrome (HS) represents an impaired sympathetic innervation of the pupil. It is characterized by unilateral miosis, ptosis, and (sometimes) ipsilateral facial anhidrosis. There are many different causes of HS. The presence of other symptoms such as facial pain, motor or coordination problems, weight loss, and diplopia helps in localization. Pharmacologic testing includes the use of cocaine eyedrops that fail to dilate the abnormal pupil. If the cocaine test is negative, pharmacologic localization can be done with hydroxyamphetamine eyedrops, which distinguish a preganglionic from a postganglionic Horner's syndrome (the pupil with a postganglionic Horner's fails to dilate). The different causes of Horner's syndrome are summarized in Table 4–3.

Once you have established that the abnormal pupil is the larger one (mydriatic), localization of the problem starts by following the course of the third nerve from the midbrain or third nerve nucleus to the iris muscle. If the problem is at the level of the midbrain, other neurologic signs are usually present (hemiparesis, nystagmus, loss of consciousness, tremor, etc.).

Third-nerve palsy is characterized by ptosis, dilated pupil, and ophthalmoplegia. Since the parasympathetic fibers run in the outer part of the third nerve and the motor fibers are more internal, compression of the

TABLE 4–2

Comparison of Visual Loss According to Localization

Lesion Level	Causes	Symptoms/Signs	Visual Field Defect
Eye	Usually refractive error; central retinal artery occlusion; retinal detachment; central retinal vein occlusion	RAPD present; usually unilateral; improves with pinhole	Depends on the cause; only one eye affected
Optic nerve	Usually inflammatory lesions (MS and sarcoid); ischemic (vasculitis, atherosclerosis), such as AION; infiltrative (neoplasia)	Monocular visual loss; ipsilateral RAPD; disc swelling	Central, centrocecal, arcuate, or wedge field defect in the affected eye
Chiasm	Parasellar mass, including pituitary adenoma, craniopharyngioma, meningioma, aneurysm, etc.	Binocular visual loss; RAPD	Bitemporal hemianopia; central scotoma and centrocecal scotoma; important to evaluate contralateral superior temporal visual field
Lateral geniculate nucleus	Infarction, neoplasia, AVM	Binocular visual loss; no RAPD	Incongruous contralateral hemianopia
Optic radiation	Infarction, inflammatory, neoplasia, AVM	Binocular visual loss; ipsilateral smooth pursuit abnormalities; spasticity of conjugate gaze; no RAPD	
Temporal lobe			Superior contralateral quadrantanopia
Parietal lobe			Inferior contralateral quadrantanopia
Occipital lobe	Infarction (PCA strokes), inflammatory, neoplasia, AVM	Binocular visual loss; no RAPD	Congruous contralateral hemianopia with macular sparing

AION, anterior ischemic optic neuropathy; PCA, posterior cerebral artery; RAPD, relative afferent pupillary defect; AVM, arteriovenous malformation.

nerve initially produces a dilated pupil without compromising eye movements. On the other hand, vascular problems producing third-nerve ischemia (diabetes) will produce a pupil-sparing third-nerve lesion, in which the pupil is normal and reactive but there is palsy of the ocular muscles innervated by the third nerve.

Tonic pupil (Adie's pupil) results from interruption of the parasympathetic supply arising from the ciliary

TABLE 4–3

Etiology of Horner's Syndrome

First-order Horner's, or central Horner's:
  Hypothalamic infarcts, tumor
  Mesencephalic stroke
  Brainstem: ischemia (Wallenberg's syndrome), tumor, hemorrhage
  Spinal cord: syringomyelias, trauma

Second-order Horner's, or preganglionic:
  Cervicothoracic cord/spinal root trauma
  Cervical spondylosis
  Pulmonary apical tumor: Pancoast tumor

Third-order Horner's, or postganglionic:
  Superior cervical ganglion (tumor, iatrogenic, etc.)
  Internal carotid artery: dissection, trauma, thrombosis, tumor, etc.
  Base of skull: tumor, trauma
  Middle ear problems
  Cavernous sinus: tumor, inflammation (Tolosa-Hunt syndrome), aneurysm, thrombosis, fistula

ganglion (cell bodies or postganglionic fibers). Symptoms include anisocoria, photophobia, and blurred near vision (because of some accommodation paresis). The exam shows a dilated pupil, poor light reaction (with the typical segmental contraction), and light-near dissociation. Clinical signs make the diagnosis. It can be confirmed by demonstrating supersensitivity of the affected pupil to 0.1% pilocarpine, which will produce more contraction in the affected pupil than in the normal pupil.

Argyll Robertson pupil is classically associated with syphilis. Usually both pupils are small and irregular, with impaired light reaction and intact near response (light-near dissociation); pupils also dilate poorly to mydriatic agents.

◆ KEY POINTS ◆

1. Horner's syndrome is characterized by ipsilateral miosis, ptosis, and ipsilateral facial anhidrosis.

2. A complete third-nerve palsy presents with mydriasis, ptosis, and ophthalmoplegia.

3. Adie's pupil is dilated, with segmental contraction and light-near dissociation.

4. Argyll Robertson pupils are small and poorly reactive to light but have preserved near response; they are typically associated with syphilis.

5. Light-near dissociation (LND): Normally the pupil constriction to light is greater than to a near stimulus. The opposite is called LND. It implies a defect in light response, such as in optic neuropathy, or the presence of aberrant regeneration, such as in Adie's pupil. Other causes of LND include dorsal midbrain lesions and severe bilateral visual loss.

Abnormal Optic Disc

The term *papilledema* implies optic disc swelling that results from increased intracranial pressure (ICP). Other forms of optic disc swelling due to local or systemic causes should just be called *optic disc swelling* (ODS).

The etiology of papilledema is a blockage of axoplasmic transport in the optic nerve. The clinical symptoms depend on the underlying etiology (pain on eye movements with demyelinating optic neuritis, sudden visual loss in anterior ischemic optic neuropathy [AION], morning headache with space-occupying lesions, etc.). The most common symptom of ODS is transient visual obscurations, described as a dimming or "blacking out" of vision, usually lasting just a few seconds. They are usually precipitated by changes in posture (bending or straightening) and can occur many times per day.

The most common causes of unilateral optic disc edema are optic neuritis, AION, and orbital compressive lesions. As a rule, optic nerve function is abnormal in each. The optic disc appearance may be indistinguishable in these entities, but certain features of the disc appearance may suggest a specific diagnosis. Disc hemorrhages, for example, are much more common in AION than in optic neuritis or compressive lesions. The *Foster-Kennedy syndrome* refers to ipsilateral optic disc atrophy due to compression by a space-occupying lesion in the frontal lobe, and papilledema in the contralateral optic disc due to increased ICP.

Table 4–4 summarizes optic disc abnormalities and describes the most relevant clinical characteristics.

◆ KEY POINTS ◆

1. Always remember to carry your ophthalmoscope.
2. An abnormal optic disc has many possible etiologies (see Table 4–4).
3. LP determines intracranial pressure.

Diplopia

Double vision usually arises from a misalignment of the eyes. It may occur from a decompensation of a previous strabismus, but in most cases it is a symptom of neurologic disease. Some of these disorders are transient and resolve spontaneously, whereas others deteriorate because of serious illness, such as stroke, tumor, multiple sclerosis, aneurysm, and systemic diseases.

Abnormal eye movements can result from disturbances at several levels: lesions in individual muscles, the neuromuscular junction, oculomotor nerves and their three paired nuclei in the brainstem, and the internuclear medial longitudinal fasciculus (MLF) that yokes the eyes in horizontal movements (Fig. 4–2). A few definitions required for understanding eye movements are summarized in Table 4–5.

Anatomy of Eye Movements

The three cranial nerves (CNs) involved in eye movements are the oculomotor (III), the trochlear (IV), and the abducens (VI). CN III innervates superior rectus, medial rectus, inferior rectus, levator palpebrae, pupil constrictor, and inferior oblique muscles. Its dysfunction produces ptosis, mydriasis, and ophthalmoparesis with the eye deviated down and out. According to the site of the lesion, there may be one of the following patterns:

- *Nucleus of CN III:* Bilateral ptosis and weakness of contralateral superior rectus

- *Subarachnoid space:* Meningismus, constitutional symptoms, and cranial nerve defects
- *Tentorial edge compression:* Depressed level of consciousness, hemiparesis, and history of trauma or supratentorial mass lesion

CN IV innervates the superior oblique muscle that intorts and depresses the adducted eye. IVth nerve lesions produce oblique diplopia, worse on downgaze when the affected eye is adducted. The patient usually complains of diplopia when reading or when going down stairs. Patients compensate with a contralateral head tilt (in other words, the diplopia improves with head tilt away from the side of the lesion).

CN VI innervates the lateral rectus muscle. Lesions produce esotropia, especially on ipsilateral gaze. VIth nerve palsy can be a nonlocalizing sign of increased ICP.

The most common causes of oculomotor nerve dysfunction in older adults include microvascular occlusion and ischemia, commonly associated with hypertension, diabetes mellitus, and atherosclerosis.

Destruction of the abducens nucleus in the brainstem leads to ipsilateral conjugate gaze palsy because of damage of the interneurons connected to the contralateral third nerve through the MLF (Fig. 4–3).

Clinical Evaluation of Diplopia

Is it monocular or binocular? If binocular, is it horizontal or vertical? Is it worse at near or far? And finally, is the problem localized to an extraocular muscle (paresis or fatigue), brainstem MLF (internuclear ophthalmoplegia), or to the orbit itself?

The MLF connects the abducens nucleus with the contralateral third-nerve nucleus (see Fig. 4–2). Lesions of the MLF produce an internuclear ophthalmoplegia (INO). The clinical characteristics of a right INO include inability to adduct the right eye in left lateral gaze plus nystagmus of the abducting left eye. Adduction during convergence is maintained because this action does not depend on the MLF. Bilateral INOs can be seen in Wernicke's encephalopathy (along with gait ataxia or confusional state), botulism, myasthenia gravis, brainstem strokes, and demyelination.

"One and a half syndrome" occurs as a consequence of a lesion involving the paramedian pontine reticular formation (PPRF) or sixth-nerve nucleus and the adjacent ipsilateral MLF. These produce an ipsilateral gaze

TABLE 4–4

Assessment of Abnormal Optic Disc

Symptom	Etiology	Clinical Manifestations	Diagnosis and Therapy	Funduscopy
Increased intracranial pressure	Space-occupying lesion (tumor, AVM, aneurysm, edema, etc.) IIH, also known as pseudotumor cerebri	Symptoms include morning headache, ataxia, and transient visual obscuration No RAPD Central acuity spared No color loss Enlarged blind spot Visual field constriction with occasional interior nasal defect	Clinical MRI/CT LP with opening pressure **Therapy:** Specific to the cause. In IIH, close follow-up of visual fields, acetazolamide, and nerve decompression	Bilateral disc hyperemia Preserved cup No VP or blurring of vessels
Drusen (calcified hyaline bodies) or pseudopapilledema	Small hyaline concretions (familial, autosomal dominant)	Asymptomatic Visual exam can demonstrate an irregular peripheral contraction Enlarged blind spot Normal visual acuity (initially)	Clinical CT and orbital ultrasound to see calcified hyaline bodies	Glistening hyaline bodies + VP Disc with irregular nodular appearance No disc hyperemia, no hemorrhage or exudates Irregular disc border and absent cup
Optic neuritis	Usually indicates demyelination (MS, lupus, adrenoleukodystrophy, sarcoid, and tumor)	Painful visual loss Uhthoff's phenomenon (worsening visual function during exercise, hot baths, etc.)	Clinical MRI looking for demyelination LP Visual evoked potentials	Variable From normal to optic atrophy Papillitis (optic nerve elevation) with optic disc swelling

	Viral—like rubella, herpes zoster, mumps	Other systemic signs of demyelination	**Therapy:** IV methylprednisolone. If MRI of the head shows more than 3 demyelinating lesions, the probability of developing MS is up to 50% in 5 years.	
	Inflammatory: meningitis, cysticercosis, etc.	Photopsias		
	Associated with systemic disease: Behçet's, Whipple's, Crohn's	Retro-orbital pain		
		RAPD		
		Loss of color discrimination		
		Central scotoma is classic		
Ischemia (AION)	Vascular: carotid occlusion, embolic TIAs	Sudden painless visual loss	Medical w/u for diabetes, hypertension, vasculitis	Usually unilateral segmental disc edema
		Patients usually older than 50		
	Inflammatory: temporal arteritis	Hypertension and diabetes associated	MRA or carotid ultrasound of the carotid artery	Possible contralateral absent cup
		Hypotensive episodes	TIA w/u	
		Exam shows variable visual field abnormalities	**Therapy:** Depends on the cause	
		RAPD is common		

IIH, idiopathic intracranial hypertension; AVM, arteriovenous malformation; RAPD, relative afferent pupillary defect; MRI, magnetic resonance imaging; CT, computed tomography; LP, lumbar puncture; VP, venous pulsation; MS, multiple sclerosis; AION, anterior ischemic optic neuropathy; TIA, transient ischemic attack; w/u, workup; MRA, magnetic resonance arteriography.

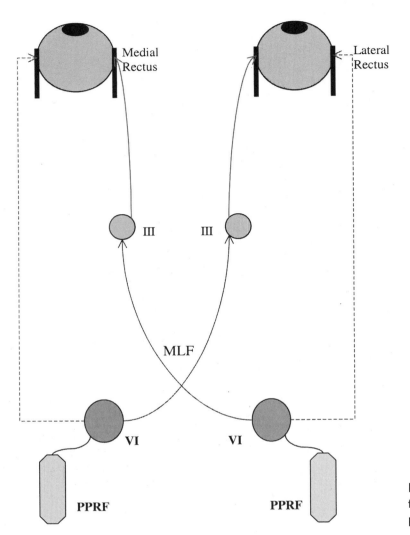

Figure 4–2 Medial longitudinal fasciculus (MLF). PPRF, paramedian pontine reticular formation.

TABLE 4–5

Some Terms Used to Define Eye Misalignment

Strabismus	Misalignment of the eyes
Comitant	Misalignment is constant in all the directions of gaze, and each eye has full range of movement (usually an ophthalmologic problem)
Noncomitant	The degree of misalignment varies with the direction of gaze (usually a neurologic problem)
Phoria	Misalignment of the eyes when binocular vision is absent
Tropia	Misalignment of the eyes when both eyes are opened and binocular vision is possible

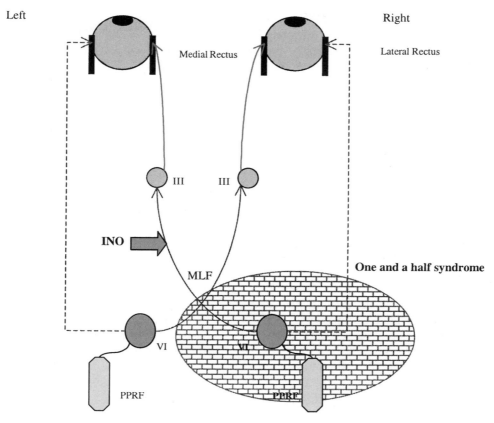

Figure 4–3 Damage to the paramedian pontine reticular formation (PPRF), VI nerve nucleus, and both medial longitudinal fasciculi (MLF) produces the one and a half syndrome (square-patterned circle). The only eye movement present in the horizontal plane in this case is the abduction of the left eye. Internuclear ophthalmoplegia (INO) occurs after damage of the MLF. In this graphic, damage to the left MLF produces inability to adduct the left eye and nystagmus in the right eye with right lateral gaze.

palsy and INO on the contralateral side (the only eye movement present in the lateral plane is abduction of the contralateral eye) (see Fig. 4–3).

Vertical eye movements are controlled by the rostral interstitial nucleus of the MLF (riMLF) located in the pretectal area, near the CN III nucleus. Fibers controlling upgaze from the riMLF cross to the contralateral side using the posterior commissure to communicate with the inferior oblique and superior rectus subnuclei of the CN III complex. The downgaze pathway is less understood but does not travel in the posterior commissure. Abnormal vertical gaze movements can be found in dorsal midbrain syndromes. Parinaud's syndrome is characterized by upgaze disturbance, convergence-retraction nystagmus on attempted upgaze, and light-near dissociation of the pupils, generally produced by a pineal tumor compressing the dorsal midbrain.

Finally, skew deviation is a vertical tropia generally caused by brainstem or cerebellar lesions. The hypotropic (lower) eye is often on the side of the lesion.

Diagnosis of Diplopia

The evaluation includes a careful history and a detailed neurologic exam. Some tests done to evaluate diplopia include the following.

- *Cover test:* Detects a tropia. Ask the patient to fixate on a small target. Cover one eye and watch the other eye. If the eye makes a refixation movement, this means that this eye was not aligned on the target. If the eye moves nasally, the patient has an exotropia; if it moves temporally, he has an esotropia. For example, a third-nerve palsy produces exotropia and hypotropia of the paretic eye. Abducens palsy produces esotropia of the affected eye.

- *Alternate cover test:* Detects phoria (esophoria or exophoria). Phoria do not cause diplopia because the eyes are aligned when both are opened simultaneously.

- *Park's three-step test:* Detects a fourth-nerve palsy:
  1. Hypertropia of the paretic eye.
  2. Hypertropia increases when the patient looks to the opposite side.
  3. Hypertropia increases when the patient tilts the head to the same side.

- *Oculocephalic maneuver (doll's eye test):* Useful in unconscious patients to evaluate the integrity of the vestibular and oculomotor apparatus. It is done by rapid horizontal and vertical movements of the head. The vestibulo-ocular reflex rotates the eyes in the opposite direction of head movement.

- *Saccades:* Rapid, conjugate movement of the eyes between objects (fingertips). In general, disorders of eye movements will produce slowness of saccades in the direction of the paretic muscle.

- *Pupillary size and reflexes*

- *Periocular signs or proptosis*

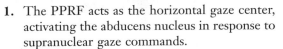

◆ KEY POINTS ◆

1. The PPRF acts as the horizontal gaze center, activating the abducens nucleus in response to supranuclear gaze commands.
2. The abducens nucleus contains motor neurons and internuclear neurons that travel with the MLF to the contralateral oculomotor nuclei in the midbrain.
3. Lesions of the MLF produce an INO.
4. Lesions of the PPRF and ipsilateral MLF produce the one and a half syndrome (gaze palsy to the ipsilateral side and INO in contralateral gaze).
5. The riMLF is the vertical gaze center, analogous to the PPRF for horizontal gaze.
6. The presence of gaze palsy may indicate a supranuclear or nuclear dysfunction. The doll's eye maneuver or caloric testing will distinguish them. If doll's eye movements are normal, the dysfunction is supranuclear.

Supranuclear Eye Movements

Saccades are rapid eye movements to redirect the eyes to a new fixation object. In general, voluntary saccades

---

TABLE 4–6

Saccadic Abnormalities

Lesion	Saccades
Unilateral cerebral	Damage contralateral saccades transiently. Bilateral parieto-occipital lesions damage visually guided saccades.
Diencephalic-mesencephalic	Impair vertical saccades. Thalamic lesions often produce downward, convergent, or contralateral eye deviation. Dorsal mesencephalic lesions preferentially impair upward gaze, and the eyes may deviate downward. Tegmental mesencephalic lesions may impair downward gaze preferentially.
Pontine	Impair horizontal saccades ipsilateral to the lesions.
Medullar and cerebellar	Cause hypometric and dysmetric saccades.

Lesions may be due to stroke, tumor, arteriovenous malformation, toxic etiologies, degenerative disease, and so forth.

TABLE 4–7

Types of Nystagmus

Type	Characteristics
Physiologic or nonpathologic	
Optokinetic nystagmus	Normal response to a continuously moving object.
Vestibulo-ocular	By rotations of the subject's head. Also irrigation of the ear (caloric test)
Endpoint nystagmus	Few beats of nystagmus in eccentric gaze.
Congenital nystagmus	Jerk or pendular, present after birth and remains throughout life.
Pathologic or acquired nystagmus	
Periodic alternating nystagmus	Horizontal jerk nystagmus that changes direction every 2–3 minutes. Acquired forms are associated with craniocervical junction abnormalities, multiple sclerosis, bilateral blindness, and toxicity from anticonvulsants.
Downbeat nystagmus	Present in primary position. Also seen in disorders of the craniocervical junction (Chiari malformation), spinocerebellar degeneration, multiple sclerosis, familial periodic ataxia, and drug intoxication.
Upbeat nystagmus	In primary position is associated with lesions of the anterior cerebellar vermis and lower brainstem. Also occurs with drug intoxication and Wernicke's encephalopathy.
See-saw nystagmus	One eye elevates and intorts while the other depresses and extorts. Associated with third ventricle tumors and bitemporal hemianopsia, trauma, and brainstem vascular disease.
Gaze-evoked nystagmus	Similar to end-point nystagmus but amplitude is greater and it occurs in a less eccentric position of the eyes. Most common cause is drug intoxication. Also seen in cerebellar disease and brainstem or hemisphere pathology.
Rebound nystagmus	Seen as a transient, rapid, horizontal jerk when eyes are moving to or from eccentric position. Usually associated with cerebellar or posterior fossa lesions.
Vestibular nystagmus	Usually horizontal with a rotatory component. Associated with peripheral inner ear disorders, Ménière's disease, vascular disorder, and drug toxicity.

originate in the frontal eye field and superior colliculus contralateral to the direction of gaze. These areas have a direct connection with the contralateral PPRF and participate in saccadic movements. Other areas that contribute to saccadic control include the dorsolateral prefrontal cortex, supplementary eye field, and parietal lobe. Vertical saccades may also originate in frontal eye fields or superior colliculi and connect to the contralateral riMLF. Inability to produce saccades is called *ocular motor apraxia*.

Abnormal saccades include those that overshoot (hypermetric) or undershoot (hypometric), and unwanted saccades or saccadic intrusions (square wave jerks, ocular flutter, and opsoclonus).

Lesions of particular brain regions are associated with specific clinical manifestations (Table 4–6).

Pursuit movements permit the eyes to conjugately track a moving visual target to keep it in focus. The control is hemispheric and ipsilateral. Visual cortex inputs reach the temporo-occipital region.

TABLE 4–8

Tips for Differentiating Central from Peripheral Nystagmus

	Peripheral (vestibular)	Central (brainstem)
Direction	Unidirectional, fast phase away from the lesion	Bidirectional or unidirectional
Purely horizontal without rotatory component	Uncommon	Common
Vertical nystagmus	Never present	May be present
Visual fixation	Inhibits nystagmus and vertigo	No changes
Tinnitus or deafness	Often present	Rarely present
Romberg signs	Toward the slow phase	Variable
Vertigo	Severe	Mild
Duration	Short but recurrent	May be chronic
Causes	Vascular disorders, trauma, toxicity, Ménière's disease, vestibular neuronitis	Vascular, demyelination, and neoplastic/ paraneoplastic disorders.

The occipito-parietal-temporal junction is responsible for integrating the movement data. The fibers course into the deep parietal lobe and continue to the ipsilateral dorsolateral pontine nucleus. Then they travel sequentially to the cerebellar vermis, nucleus prepositus hypoglossi, medial vestibular nuclei, and finally to the abducens nuclei for horizontal pursuit. Vertical pursuits are mediated by the interstitial nucleus of Cajal rather than the riMLF (as for vertical saccades).

Pursuit disorders may be difficult to identify. Neurologic diseases such as Parkinson's disease, progressive supranuclear palsy, drugs, and aging can slow down pursuits. Deep parietal lobe lesions produce pursuit abnormalities as well. Because of the long pathway involved in this type of movement, its value in localizing a lesion is limited.

The vestibulo-ocular reflex (VOR) coordinates eye movements with head movement, allowing the visual image to not slip during movements of the head. Slow passive head movements can elicit it. The pathway involves the semicircular canals (rotation) and otoliths (linear acceleration) and travels to the vestibular nuclei. From there, it proceeds to the abducens nuclei and then to cranial nerves III and IV through the MLF. Abnormalities of the VOR result in nystagmus (see the following subsection).

Nystagmus

Nystagmus is a rhythmic to-and-fro movement of the eyes. It can be either pendular or jerk. In jerk nystagmus, the eye drifts away from fixation in a pursuit-like movement and returns with a fast, saccadic movement. The direction of the nystagmus is named by the direction of this fast component.

Nystagmus may be congenital, physiologic, or a sign of CNS dysfunction, peripheral vestibular loss, or visual loss. Table 4–7 provides a brief description of physiologic and acquired nystagmus as well as the possible causes.

Special attention needs to be paid to vestibular nystagmus. It is very common to be called to the emergency room (ER) to evaluate a patient with the acute onset of vertigo; the ER doctor immediately becomes concerned when the patient has nystagmus.

Table 4–8 describes a few characteristics to help differentiate central from peripheral nystagmus.

◆ KEY POINTS ◆

1. Peripheral nystagmus is usually unidirectional, with the fast phase away from the lesion; it combines horizontal and torsional movements and is inhibited by fixation.

2. Central nystagmus is normally bidirectional, often purely horizontal, vertical, or torsional, and not inhibited by fixation.

3. Saccades are fast eye movements that redirect the fovea to a new target. Horizontal saccades are initiated in the contralateral frontal eye field or superior colliculus.

4. Vertical saccades originate from bilateral frontal eye fields or the superior colliculus.

5. Conjugate gaze deviation is observed in lesions of the frontal lobe with destruction of the frontal eye field; the eyes deviate toward the side of the lesion. During a seizure, the eyes look away from the frontal focus.

5

The Approach to Weakness

Weakness is one of the most common presenting neurologic complaints. Many patients may tolerate some degree of numbness, tingling, or even pain, but often it is when weakness sets in that medical attention is finally sought. Similarly, friends or family members will not notice a patient's sensory problems, but significant weakness will be obvious to all.

At the same time, weakness can be one of the most difficult neurologic problems to sort out, because the pathways that control motor function span the entire axis of the nervous system. Left leg weakness can arise from a peripheral nerve lesion, a lumbosacral plexus problem, or a stroke in the right cerebral hemisphere: Each of these has a different workup, prognosis, and treatment, and it is the job of the physician to use the history and examination to distinguish among them.

PRINCIPLES

Figure 5–1 presents a flowchart to aid in the diagnosis of weakness. The key steps in the clinical approach are outlined below.

1. *Make sure that true weakness is the complaint.* Sometimes patients will use the term *weak* to mean a general sense of fatigue; others will say a limb is "weak" when it is clumsy or numb. Having the patient confirm that decreased strength is the symptom may be useful. Likewise, a limb that is painful to move may seem

"weak"; whether there is true underlying weakness may be difficult to discern.

2. *Identify which muscles are weak.* This seems like an obvious point but must be emphasized. It is not sufficient to know that a patient has left leg weakness. Testing must be done in enough detail to know which muscles in the left leg are weak or, if they are all diffusely weak, which are weaker than others.

3. *Determine the pattern of weakness.* This is frequently the crux of the entire diagnosis. It is the pattern of weakness that will reveal when left leg weakness is due to a peroneal nerve problem and not a right hemisphere stroke. Needless to say, one must be familiar with the different patterns of weakness and their implications.

4. *Look for associated signs and symptoms.* If a leg is weak, determine whether it is also numb, tingling, or painful. Check the reflexes carefully. Often the motor deficit overshadows other problems whose presence may be helpful in supporting or excluding certain diagnoses.

5. *Use laboratory and electrophysiologic tests wisely.* Blood tests or neuroimaging studies can be useful in the appropriate settings, and electromyography/nerve conduction studies (EMG/NCS) can act as an extension of the clinical exam in localizing the problem to a particular segment of the peripheral nervous system. Tests are most useful in the setting of a complete clinical evaluation and formed diagnostic hypothesis, however.

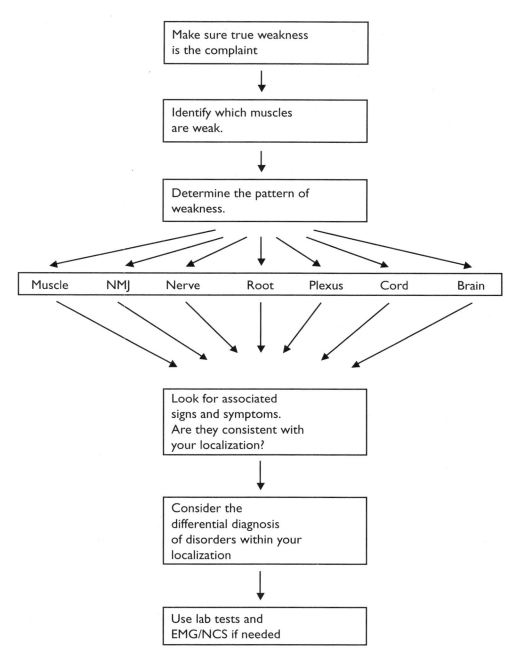

Figure 5–1　The approach to weakness.

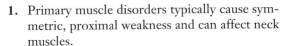

◆ KEY POINTS ◆

1. Weakness can be caused by lesions along the entire neuraxis, from brain to muscle.

2. The diagnosis rests on determining what the pattern of weakness is, searching for associated signs and symptoms, and using laboratory tests and EMG/NCS to confirm clinical hypotheses.

DIFFERENTIAL DIAGNOSIS OF WEAKNESS

It is useful to consider the disorders that cause weakness in an anatomic order, from most distal in the nervous system (primary muscle disorders) to most proximal (disorders of the cerebral hemisphere). Below, each anatomic category is presented with the clues that might lead a clinician to suspect a disorder in that location. Individual diseases in each category are discussed in the later chapters covering specific neurologic disorders.

Primary Muscle Disorders

Pattern of Weakness
Primary muscle problems tend to cause weakness predominantly in proximal muscles, in a symmetric fashion. Distal muscles are affected later or not as severely. In addition, neck flexors and extensors, which are not affected in most nerve or brain lesions, may be weak in a muscle disorder.

Associated Signs and Symptoms
Associated signs and symptoms may occasionally include muscle pain if the muscle disorder is inflammatory, such as polymyositis. By their nature, primary disorders of muscle should not cause other sensory signs or symptoms. Reflexes are characteristically preserved, unless the process is so severe that the muscles are nearly paralyzed.

Laboratory Studies
Some disorders of muscle are characterized by an elevated serum creatine kinase (CK) level. The demonstration of characteristic "myopathic" changes on an EMG can help confirm a primary muscle disorder.

Differential Diagnosis
Primary muscle disorders, discussed in Chapter 24, include both acquired problems (myopathies), which can result from inflammatory or toxic etiologies, among other causes, and congenital problems (muscular dystrophies).

◆ KEY POINTS ◆

1. Primary muscle disorders typically cause symmetric, proximal weakness and can affect neck muscles.

2. Sensory signs and symptoms are not present.

3. Serum CK level is elevated in some muscle disorders, and EMG may show a characteristic "myopathic" pattern.

Neuromuscular Junction Disorders

Pattern of Weakness
Neuromuscular junction (NMJ) problems can vary in the pattern of weakness they cause, though most affect proximal extremity muscles. Some NMJ disorders can lead to ptosis as well as weakness of extraocular, bulbar, and neck muscles. The characteristic feature of NMJ disorders is not the pattern of weakness, however, but the fluctuation. The degree of weakness may change from hour to hour. Depending on the specific disease, strength may be worse after using the muscles or toward the end of the day, and improve after resting or in the morning (fatigability). Alternatively, strength may paradoxically improve after exercise in other conditions.

Associated Signs and Symptoms
By their nature, NMJ problems, which affect only the junction between the motor axon terminal and the muscle, should not lead to sensory signs or symptoms. Some NMJ disorders may have associated autonomic features.

Laboratory Studies
EMG/NCS can demonstrate nearly pathognomonic findings for certain NMJ disorders on specialized testing. Some of the diseases in this category have specific serum markers, such as anti-acetylcholine receptor antibodies in myasthenia gravis.

Differential Diagnosis
NMJ disorders are discussed in Chapter 24 and include myasthenia gravis and Lambert-Eaton myasthenic syndrome, among others.

◆ KEY POINTS ◆

1. NMJ disorders can cause weakness of proximal muscles; some characteristically affect extraocular and bulbar muscles.

2. The key to diagnosing NMJ disorders is fluctuation in the degree of weakness.

3. Sensory signs and symptoms are not present.

4. EMG/NCS can be nearly pathognomonic in some cases.

Peripheral Nerve Disorders

Pattern of Weakness

Each muscle in the upper or lower extremity is innervated by a named peripheral nerve (Table 5–1). A lesion involving a particular peripheral nerve will lead to weakness in the muscles innervated by that nerve, while sparing other, often neighboring, muscles.

Disorders affecting a single peripheral nerve are known as *mononeuropathies*. Certain systemic conditions can lead to dysfunction of multiple peripheral nerves in succession, a disorder known as *mononeuropathy multiplex*. Finally, when peripheral nerves are all affected diffusely, in a *polyneuropathy*, dysfunction typically occurs in the longest nerves first. Thus, weakness from

TABLE 5–1

Commonly Tested Movements

Movement	Muscle	Nerve	Root
Shoulder abduction	Deltoid	Axillary	C5
Elbow flexion	Biceps	Musculocutaneous	C5/C6
Elbow extension	Triceps	Radial	C7
Wrist extension	Wrist extensors	Radial	C7
Finger flexion	Finger flexors	Median, ulnar	C8/T1
Finger extension	Finger extensors	Radial	C7
Finger abduction	Interossei	Ulnar	C8/T1
Hip flexion	Iliopsoas	Nerve to iliopsoas	L1/L2/L3
Hip abduction	Gluteus medius, minimus	Superior gluteal	L5
Hip adduction	Hip adductors	Obturator	L2/L3
Hip extension	Gluteus maximus	Sciatic	S1
Knee flexion	Hamstrings	Sciatic	L5/S1
Knee extension	Quadriceps	Femoral	L3/L4
Plantarflexion	Gastrocnemius, soleus	Tibial	S1
Dorsiflexion	Tibialis anterior	Peroneal	L5
Eversion	Peroneus muscles	Peroneal	S1
Inversion	Tibialis posterior	Tibial	L5
Great toe extension	Extensor hallucis longus	Peroneal	L5

a polyneuropathy usually appears first in the distal muscles, symmetrically.

Associated Signs and Symptoms

Mononeuropathies may have sensory symptoms, such as numbness, tingling, or pain, in the distribution of the relevant peripheral nerve. Mononeuropathy multiplex is characteristically associated with pain. Polyneuropathies, depending on etiology, usually have associated sensory loss and depressed or absent reflexes, particularly in the distal extremities.

Laboratory Studies

EMG/NCS can confirm the clinical suspicion of a problem localized to the peripheral nerves. NCS can identify whether the pathologic process affects primarily the axons or the myelin of the nerve, an essential step in formulating a differential diagnosis. EMG may yield insight as to the relative acuity or chronicity of a nerve disorder.

Differential Diagnosis

Mononeuropathies most commonly occur as a result of entrapment (as in carpal tunnel syndrome). Mononeuropathy multiplex is associated with systemic vasculitis and other metabolic or rheumatologic diseases. Demyelinating polyneuropathies can be hereditary (such as Charcot-Marie-Tooth) or acquired (as in Guillain-Barré), while axonal polyneuropathies have many potential underlying causes. Peripheral nerve disorders are discussed in Chapter 23.

◆ KEY POINTS ◆

1. Mononeuropathies lead to weakness in muscles innervated by a single peripheral nerve.
2. Polyneuropathies first affect the distal extremity muscles symmetrically.
3. EMG/NCS can confirm peripheral nerve involvement, identify axonal or demyelinating features, and evaluate the relative chronicity of a nerve disorder.

Nerve Root Disorders

Pattern of Weakness

Each nerve root relevant to the upper or lower extremity exits the spinal cord and eventually traverses a plexus

(either brachial or lumbosacral) in which its fibers separate and become part of multiple different peripheral nerves, which then go on to innervate multiple different muscles. The result is that most muscles are innervated by fibers that originate from more than one nerve root, although some muscles are predominantly innervated by fibers from one nerve root (see Table 5–1). In any case, a lesion of a single nerve root will cause weakness in the muscles innervated predominantly by fibers from that root, while leaving other, often neighboring, muscles unaffected.

A single nerve root problem is termed a *radiculopathy*. Some processes lead to dysfunction of multiple nerve roots at once (*polyradiculopathy*), leaving a pattern of weakness that may be diffuse and difficult to sort out because multiple muscles related to multiple nerve roots can be weak bilaterally.

Associated Signs and Symptoms

Radiculopathies often have associated tingling or pain, frequently radiating out from the neck or back. Objective sensory loss is rare in disorders affecting a single nerve root, because there is overlap from neighboring roots. If the nerve root is one that subserves a particular muscle stretch reflex (Table 5–2), that reflex may be depressed or absent.

Laboratory Studies

EMG/NCS can confirm that nerve roots are the culprit in a weak patient, and can be particularly useful for cases in which clinical differentiation between a root problem and a peripheral nerve problem is murky. Single radiculopathies usually require magnetic resonance imaging

---

TABLE 5–2

Commonly Tested Muscle Stretch Reflexes

Reflex	Root
Biceps	C5
Brachioradialis	C6
Triceps	C7
Finger flexor	C8/T1
Patellar (knee jerk)	L4
Hip adductor	L3
Ankle jerk	S1

(MRI) of the spine to rule out structural etiologies, whereas polyradiculopathies usually require lumbar puncture (LP) to look for infectious or inflammatory conditions.

Differential Diagnosis

Single radiculopathies can be caused by herniated discs or by reactivation of varicella-zoster virus (shingles), for example. Polyradiculopathies are often inflammatory or infectious. These disorders are discussed in Chapter 23.

◆ KEY POINTS ◆

1. A radiculopathy causes weakness in the muscles innervated predominantly by fibers from one nerve root.

2. Radiating pain and tingling are common symptoms.

3. If the nerve root subserves a particular muscle stretch reflex, that reflex may be depressed or absent.

4. A polyradiculopathy may lead to weakness of multiple muscles related to multiple nerve roots bilaterally.

Plexus Disorders

Pattern of Weakness

The intricacies of brachial and lumbosacral plexus anatomy (Fig. 5–2) are often quite intimidating for students, but need not be, because ironically it is the complex anatomy that makes localizing lesions to a plexus more straightforward than expected. Put simply, if multiple muscles in a limb are weak and do not conform to the pattern of a particular nerve root or peripheral nerve, a plexus problem should be suspected.

In the leg, for example, weakness in both hip flexors and hip adductors would have to involve L1, L2, and L3 roots or both the nerve to the iliopsoas and the obturator nerve (see Table 5–1); a much more likely explanation is a lesion in the upper part of the lumbosacral plexus.

Associated Signs and Symptoms

Because the plexus is where multiple nerve roots intermingle their fibers to form multiple peripheral nerves, it is unsurprising that plexus disorders can have associated sensory findings (in the distribution of one or more roots or nerves) or dropped reflexes (subserved by one or more roots).

Laboratory Studies

EMG/NCS is frequently ordered in cases of clinically suspected plexopathies to help confirm the localization

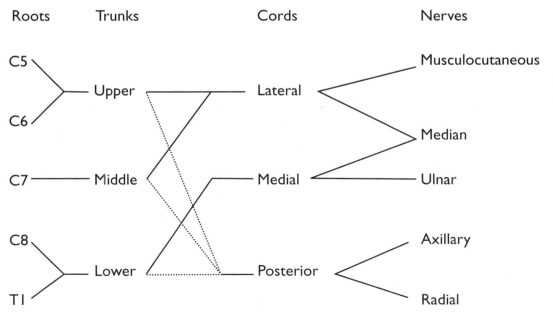

Figure 5–2 Brachial plexus anatomy.

to the plexus, given the less-than-straightforward anatomy. MRI of the brachial plexus or pelvis (or lumbosacral plexus) may be necessary to rule out mass lesions.

Differential Diagnosis

Plexopathies can be caused by idiopathic inflammation, radiation, infiltration by metastases, hemorrhage, or trauma. They are discussed in Chapter 23. Diabetic patients are prone to a characteristic lumbosacral plexopathy known as *diabetic amyotrophy*.

◆ KEY POINTS ◆

1. A plexus problem should be suspected when multiple muscles in a limb are weak and do not conform to a particular nerve root or peripheral nerve pattern.

2. There may be associated sensory signs or reflex loss.

3. Plexopathies can be confirmed by EMG/NCS and have many potential causes.

Spinal Cord Disorders

Pattern of Weakness

Spinal cord disorders cause weakness in two ways. First, the anterior horn cells located at the level of the lesion are affected, leading to weakness of the muscles innervated by the nerve root at that level. This mimics a radiculopathy, with weakness in a particular nerve root pattern. Second, there is weakness below the level of the lesion due to interruption of the descending corticospinal tracts. This weakness occurs in an upper motor neuron (UMN) pattern (Fig. 5–3).

Associated Signs and Symptoms

Depending on the extent of the lesion, there may be sensory findings due to interruption of the ascending tracts. There may be a sensory level (loss of sensation below a particular dermatomal level) on the torso. Typically, reflexes below the level of a spinal cord lesion are increased, and there may be Babinski signs. Bladder and bowel incontinence may occur.

Laboratory Studies

MRI of the spine can rule out structural etiologies or demonstrate intrinsic inflammation within the cord. LP

may be needed to evaluate infectious or inflammatory possibilities.

Differential Diagnosis

Spinal cord disorders are discussed in Chapter 22, and may stem from inflammation (transverse myelitis), infarction, compression, or other causes. Amyotrophic lateral sclerosis causes degeneration of both the corticospinal tracts and anterior horn cells.

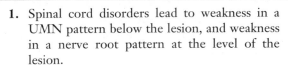

◆ KEY POINTS ◆

1. Spinal cord disorders lead to weakness in a UMN pattern below the lesion, and weakness in a nerve root pattern at the level of the lesion.

2. There may be sensory loss below the level of the lesion due to interruption of ascending tracts.

3. Reflexes below the level of the lesion are typically increased, and Babinski signs may be present.

4. Bladder and bowel incontinence may occur.

Disorders of the Cerebral Hemispheres and Brainstem

Pattern of Weakness

Lesions in the cerebral hemispheres lead to weakness of the contralateral body in a UMN pattern (see Fig. 5–3). Knowledge of the homunculus of the motor strip (Fig. 5–4) explains why lesions in the parasagittal part of the cerebral hemisphere cause weakness primarily in the leg, whereas lesions more laterally in the hemisphere cause weakness primarily in the face and arm. Deep hemisphere lesions, such as in the internal capsule, may lead to weakness of all three parts of the contralateral body (face, arm, and leg), since motor fibers from all areas of the motor strip join together as they travel toward the brainstem.

Lesions in the base of the pons may lead to weakness of the ipsilateral face and contralateral arm and leg (crossed signs), because descending motor fibers to the face have crossed at that level but those to the body have not.

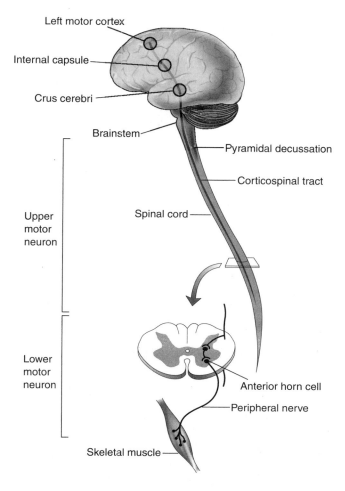

The descending motor pathway is divided into two parts.

The Upper Motor Neuron	The Lower Motor Neuron
Constitutes the neuron in the motor strip of the cerebral hemisphere and its descending axon all the way through the pyramidal decussation into the spinal cord	Constitutes the anterior horn cell and its projecting axon all the way through the root and nerve to the neuromuscular junction of the innervated muscle
Disorders of the UMN lead to a particular pattern of weakness: In the upper extremity, extensors and abductors become weaker than flexors and adductors. In the lower extremity, muscles that shorten the leg become weaker than muscles that lengthen the leg. In addition, UMN lesions lead to associated signs such as spasticity, hyperactive reflexes, and Babinski signs.	Disorders of the LMN lead to associated signs such as wasting and fasciculations.
In the face, lesions in the UMN (motor strip in cerebral hemisphere down to decussation in the pons) lead to weakness of the lower face but not the upper face, and weakness with volitional movements but not with emotional smile.	In the face, lesions in the LMN (peripheral facial nerve, as in Bell's palsy), lead to weakness of the upper and lower face, seen with all movements.

Figure 5–3 Upper motor neuron (UMN) versus lower motor neuron (LMN).

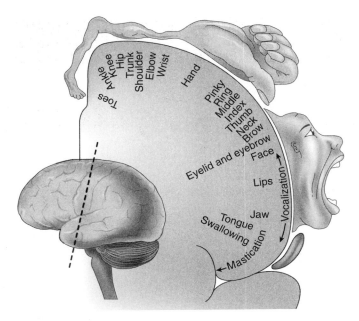

Figure 5–4 The homunculus of the motor strip.

Associated Signs and Symptoms

Lesions of the cerebral hemispheres frequently have associated cognitive signs, such as those described in Chapter 11. Left hemisphere lesions may cause aphasia or apraxia, while right hemisphere lesions may cause neglect or visuospatial dysfunction. Lesions of the brainstem may cause cranial nerve problems, such as extraocular movement disorders.

Laboratory Studies

Imaging of the brain is important to evaluate almost all of the potential etiologies in this category. The choice of MRI or computed tomography (CT) depends on the suspected etiology and relative acuity.

Differential Diagnosis

The differential diagnosis includes such diverse etiologies as stroke (Chapter 14), demyelinating disease (Chapter 20), traumatic injury (Chapter 17), brain tumor (Chapter 19), and infection (Chapter 21).

◆ KEY POINTS ◆

1. Cerebral hemisphere lesions lead to weakness of the contralateral side in a UMN pattern.

2. Parasagittal lesions lead primarily to leg weakness, more lateral lesions lead primarily to face and arm weakness, and deep lesions may lead to weakness of all three parts.

3. Cerebral hemisphere lesions may have accompanying cognitive signs, such as aphasia or neglect.

4. Brainstem lesions may have accompanying cranial nerve findings.

6

The Sensory System

The sensory system places the individual in relationship to the environment. The different modalities of sensation include somatosensory and special senses: smell, vision, taste, hearing, and vestibular sensation. All sensory systems include a receptor and afferent nerves, individual types of nerve fibers situated in the dorsal root ganglion or cranial nerve ganglion that carry the information to the central nervous system.

Abnormalities of somatosensory perception are common. They may be characterized by increase, alteration, impairment, or loss of feeling. Approach to the diagnosis of these problems includes analysis of the nature, location, characteristics, and distribution of symptoms.

ANATOMY OF THE SENSORY PATHWAYS

Each sensory modality has a receptor. The information is then carried to the central nervous system by individual fibers in the nerve (peripheral or cranial) known as first-order neurons. Pain and temperature are carried by thinly myelinated and unmyelinated slowly conducting fibers (A-delta and C) that synapse at the level of the dorsal horn of the spinal cord. From here, the axons from the second-order neurons cross and travel contralaterally in the spinothalamic tract (STT) or antero-

lateral system (Fig. 6–1). Proprioception, vibration, and light touch run ipsilaterally in heavily myelinated fibers (A-alpha and A-beta) in the dorsal column system, reaching the second-order neuron at the level of the medulla in the nuclei gracilis and cuneatus. Axons from these nuclei cross at the lower medulla to form the medial lemniscus (Fig. 6–2).

There is a somatotopic arrangement of fibers in these tracts.

- *STT:* At the level of the spinal cord, sacral segments are located laterally, lumbar fibers more medially, and cervical segments in the most medial locations.
- *The dorsal columns:* The medial fibers are from the legs; lateral fibers from the arms. At the level of the medial lemniscus, the upper body becomes medial and the lower body lateral.

Facial sensation is carried to the brainstem by the trigeminal nerve. The STT and the trigeminal tract terminate in the thalamus (ventroposterolateral and ventroposteromedial, respectively), with further cortical projections through the third-order neurons to the postcentral cortex in a somatotopic arrangement similar to the motor cortex, with the face in the lowest area and the leg in the parasagittal area. Fine sensory discrimination and localization of pain, temperature, touch, and pressure require normal functioning of the sensory cortex.

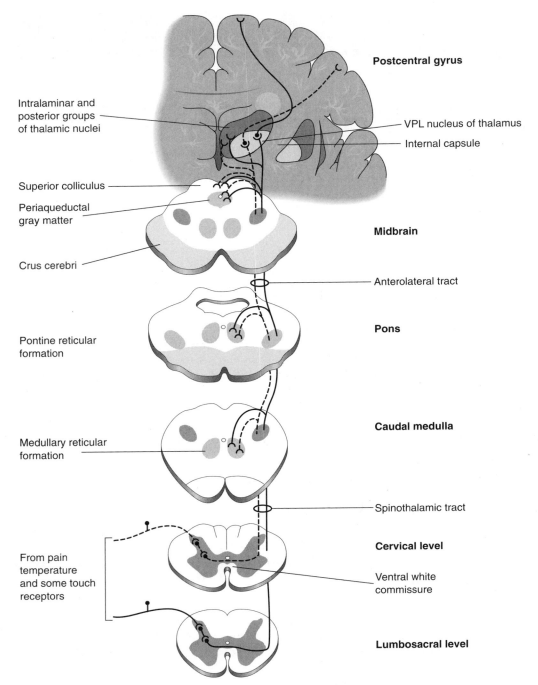

Postcentral gyrus

Intralaminar and posterior groups of thalamic nuclei

VPL nucleus of thalamus

Internal capsule

Superior colliculus

Periaqueductal gray matter

Midbrain

Crus cerebri

Anterolateral tract

Pons

Pontine reticular formation

Caudal medulla

Medullary reticular formation

Spinothalamic tract

Cervical level

From pain temperature and some touch receptors

Ventral white commissure

Lumbosacral level

Figure 6–1   Anterolateral system. VPL, ventroposterolateral.

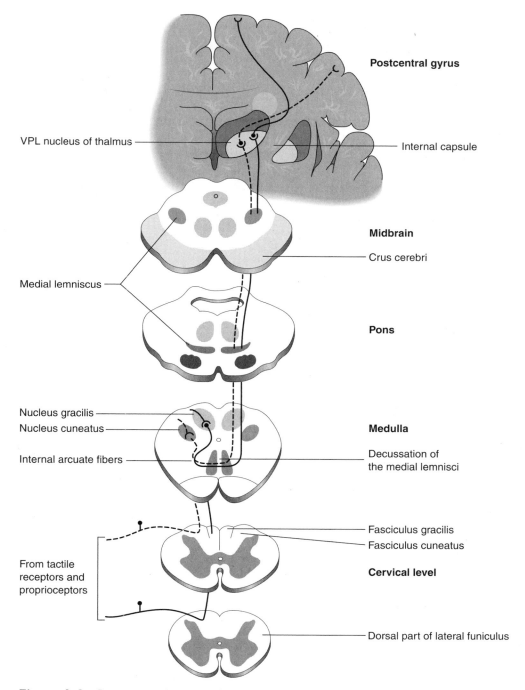

Postcentral gyrus

VPL nucleus of thalmus

Internal capsule

Midbrain

Crus cerebri

Medial lemniscus

Pons

Nucleus gracilis

Nucleus cuneatus

Medulla

Internal arcuate fibers

Decussation of
the medial lemnisci

Fasciculus gracilis

Fasciculus cuneatus

From tactile
receptors and
proprioceptors

Cervical level

Dorsal part of lateral funiculus

Figure 6–2 Posterior column–medial lemniscal system. VPL, ventroposterolateral.

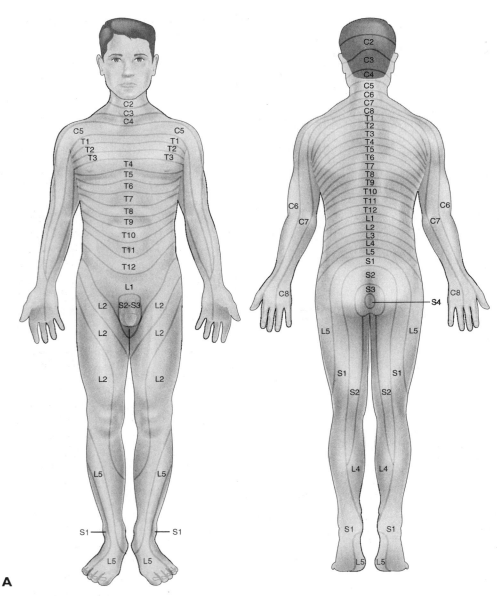

A

Figure 6–3 Dermatome map.

EXAMINATION OF THE SENSORY SYSTEM

This is a difficult part of the neurologic exam and requires the patient's alertness, intelligence, and willingness to cooperate. It is necessary to examine each sensory modality independently and use that information to better characterize the sensory loss and its extent, and the quality of the sensory deficit. Sometimes, it is difficult to demonstrate sensory abnormalities in a patient with sensory symptoms. Correspondingly, there are sometimes sensory findings in patients who

Area innervated by
trigeminal nerve (V)

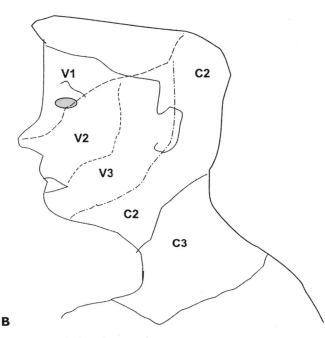

B

Figure 6–3   *Continued*

have no sensory symptoms. No matter which is the case, the sensory examination needs to be methodic and organized.

Touch sensation is tested with a wisp of cotton, using a very soft stimulus. Pain sensation is tested with a pin. Thermal modalities are tested using objects with a temperature range between 10°C and 50°C, because beyond those limits the stimulus becomes painful. Joint position sense is tested by moving the great toe up and down and asking the patient to indicate the direction of movement. You can do the same with the fingers. Proprioception can also be tested by moving an object up or down on the skin and asking the patient the direction of the movement. Vibration sense needs a tuning fork (128 Hz) applied to toes and other bony prominences.

Once you have examined the patient, the next step is to record the sensory abnormalities using accepted definitions.

It is important to register the patient's own words rather than using some of the terms described below. Not only the presence or absence of sensation, but also slight differences and gradations should be recorded.

The following list defines some of the terminology used to describe sensory abnormalities:

- *Paresthesias* mean abnormal sensations described by the patient as tingling, prickling, pins and needles, etc.
- *Dysesthesias* refer to unpleasant sensations triggered by painless stimuli.
- *Hyperesthesia* indicates increased sensitivity to sensory stimuli. The opposite is *hypesthesia*.
- *Allodynia* is used to indicate pain provoked by normally innocuous stimuli.
- *Dissociated sensory loss* refers to the loss of one of the sensory systems with preservation of another one. For example, in syrinx the STT is compromised early, with loss of pain and temperature in the dermatomes involved but preservation of posterior column function and therefore normal light touch and proprioception. This occurs frequently with central cord syndromes.

APPROACH TO THE PATIENT WITH SENSORY LOSS

Sensory dysfunction becomes manifest through two type of symptoms: *negative*, such as numbness, loss of cold or warm sensation, blindness, and deafness; or *positive*, such as pain, paresthesias (tingling, pins and needles), visual sparkles, and tinnitus. The former usually means disruption of nerve excitation; the latter in general means excitation or disinhibition.

In a patient complaining of sensory disturbances, the first goal is to establish the presence or absence of a neurologic lesion, and then establish its location. Sometimes, the sensory problems accompany other symptoms, such as weakness, neglect, visual field cuts, behavioral problems, and seizures, which help improve the localization.

The goal is to recognize sensory abnormalities by modality and to judge the level at which they are produced. Although in theory it is easy to recognize peripheral nerve from segmental nerve or root, spinal cord, or other central nervous system locations, it is in fact often not possible or at best imprecise. In general, compression of a peripheral nerve has a distribution of sensory loss in the territory of that specific nerve. Root problems give a dermatomal pattern of loss (Fig. 6–3). Spinal cord disease has a characteristic loss of sensation below

TABLE 6–1

Patterns of Sensory Loss According to Localization

Site of the Lesion	Sensory Findings	Other Neurologic Abnormalities	Examples
Peripheral nerve	Loss of LT, T, PP, and proprioception in the influenced area; associated weakness in muscles innervated by that nerve	Distal muscle weakness, atrophy, areflexia	Peroneal neuropathy; median and ulnar neuropathies
Root	Loss of all sensory modalities in a dermatomal distribution	Weakness in a myotomal distribution, atrophy, segmental hyporeflexia	L5 radiculopathy; cervical radiculopathy
Plexus	Sensory loss in the distribution of two or more peripheral nerves	Muscle weakness that cannot be localized to a single nerve or root	Brachial plexopathy due to trauma, inflammation, infiltration, etc.
Spinal cord	Sensory level: bilateral loss of all sensory modalities. Sensory dissociation. Contralateral hypesthesia and ipsilateral loss of proprioception (Brown-Séquard syndrome). Proprioceptive loss and corticospinal tract involvement. Saddle anesthesia	Paraplegia, tetraplegia; initially areflexia, then hyperreflexia below the lesion; Babinski sign	Myelopathy; central cord syndromes; Brown-Séquard syndrome; subacute combined degeneration
Brainstem	Ipsilateral facial numbness and contralateral body numbness	Alternating hemiplegia; cranial nerve findings; INO, ataxia	Posterior circulation strokes; tumor
Thalamus	Hemibody anesthesia	May have motor findings	Lacunar stroke; hemorrhage
Posterior limb of internal capsule	Hemibody anesthesia	Hemiplegia	Lacunar stroke; hemorrhage; tumor
Cortex	All modalities affected on the contralateral side	Sensory neglect; agraphesthesia	Parietal stroke; hemorrhage; AVM
Psychogenic	Hyperesthesia for one modality in one area with anesthesia for another modality in the same area; changing sensory findings. Nonphysiologic sensory level changes (abrupt midline changes, vibration asymmetry over the forehead, etc.)	Any	Psychogenic (This is a diagnosis of exclusion; all the previous causes need to be excluded before reaching this conclusion.)

LT, light touch; T, temperature; PP, pinprick; INO, internuclear ophthalmoplegia; AVM, arteriovenous malformation.

a certain level. In brainstem lesions, the sensory abnormalities may occur on the ipsilateral side of the face and contralateral side of the body. Central sensory loss involving thalamus or sensory cortex will generally affect the contralateral face, arm, and leg.

Once you have characterized the location of the sensory loss, it is important to determine what sensory modality is involved, because different pathologic processes can affect different sensory systems.

The last step in evaluating these sensory abnormalities is to establish the cause. There are many primary neurologic diseases as well as systemic diseases that can present with sensory symptoms. They are explored in more detail in the chapter on peripheral neuropathies.

The different patterns of sensory loss and the location of the neurologic problem are represented in Table 6–1. This will guide you through the process of diagnoses based on the clinical symptoms and physical exam, without the need for further technological resources.

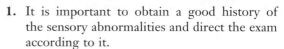

◆ KEY POINTS ◆

1. It is important to obtain a good history of the sensory abnormalities and direct the exam according to it.

2. Nerve damage produces sensory problems in the distribution of that nerve, root damage produces sensory problems in a dermatome, and plexus damage produces sensory problems in a group of nerves in the same extremity.

3. Spinal cord lesions produce a sensory level; brainstem lesions cause a crossed sensory loss; and thalamus and cortex lesions produce sensory loss in the contralateral face, arm, and leg.

7

Vertigo and Dizziness

"Dizziness" means different things to different people. Broadly speaking, the possibilities include vertigo, light-headedness, dysequilibrium, and a fourth category of ill-defined dizziness. Vertigo refers to an illusion or hallucination of movement that is usually rotatory, but may be linear. The symptom of light-headedness may also be described as feeling faint and refers to the presyncopal state. This chapter focuses on these two categories.

Dysequilibrium is a sensation of imbalance or unsteadiness that is usually referable to the legs rather than to a feeling inside the head. The pathology responsible for this symptom is outlined in detail in Chapter 8. Finally, there is the ill-defined category that includes people who simply cannot define their symptoms accurately, as well as people with anxiety.

VERTIGO

Most vertigo is caused by an acute asymmetry of neural activity between the left and right vestibular nuclei. Vertigo does not result from a slow unilateral loss of vestibular function (e.g., acoustic neuroma) or from symmetric bilateral loss of function (e.g., ototoxic drugs). A useful approach (Table 7–1) to sorting out the etiology is to determine the periodicity and duration of the symptoms, and whether they are positional or spontaneous. A determination should also be made whether the vertigo is of peripheral or central origin; the most

helpful features in this regard are the presence and nature of the associated symptoms and signs. The presence of tinnitus or hearing loss suggests a peripheral cause, whereas diplopia, dysarthria, dysphagia, or other symptoms of brainstem dysfunction indicate a central process. Accompanying nausea and vomiting is often more prominent with peripheral causes of vertigo, and the ability to walk or maintain posture may be more impaired with central pathology. Neither of these latter features, however, is very reliable. Finally, the nature of the nystagmus may suggest the source of the vertigo. Vertical and direction-changing gaze-evoked nystagmus indicate a central process. Unidirectional nystagmus may arise from either central or peripheral dysfunction.

Vestibular neuronitis presents as an acute unilateral (complete or incomplete) peripheral vestibulopathy. The designation *neuronitis* is inaccurate because there is no evidence of inflammation, but the term is retained here because of its common usage. Patients develop sudden and spontaneous onset of vertigo, nausea, and vomiting. The onset is usually over minutes to hours; symptoms peak within 24 hours and then improve gradually over several days or weeks. Complete recovery may not occur for several months. Nystagmus is strictly unilateral and may be suppressed by visual fixation. Recovery represents central compensation for the loss of peripheral vestibular function.

Labyrinthine concussion may result from head injury irrespective of whether there is an associated skull

TABLE 7–1

Approach to the Patient with Vertigo

Spontaneous vertigo
  Single prolonged episode
    Vestibular neuronitis
    Labyrinthine concussion
    Lateral medullary or cerebellar infarction
  Recurrent episodes
    Ménière's disease
    Perilymph fistula
    Migraine
    Posterior circulation ischemia
Positional vertigo
  Peripheral
    Benign positional paroxysmal vertigo (BPPV)
  Central

fracture. Vertigo is sometimes accompanied by hearing loss and tinnitus.

Infarction of labyrinth, brainstem, or cerebellum. The blood supply to the central and peripheral vestibular apparatus and the cerebellum is via the vertebrobasilar system (posterior and inferior cerebellar arteries and the superior cerebellar artery). Blood supply to the inner ear is via the internal auditory artery, a branch of the anterior inferior cerebellar artery. Infarction of the inner ear presents with sudden onset of deafness or vertigo or both.

Brainstem or cerebellar stroke is the most important differential diagnosis in patients with suspected acute vestibular neuronitis. The type of nystagmus and the presence of associated neurologic signs are the main distinguishing factors. A central-type nystagmus results from cerebellar or brainstem infarction, and almost invariably there are associated cranial nerve signs, weakness, ataxia, or sensory changes that clearly indicate a central process.

Ménière's disease is characterized by episodic vertigo with nausea and vomiting; fluctuating, but progressive hearing loss; tinnitus; and a sensation of fullness or pressure in the ear. It is caused by an intermittent increase in endolymphatic volume.

A *perilymph fistula* results from disruption of the lining of the endolymphatic system. Typically, the patient reports hearing a "pop" at the time of a sudden increase in middle ear pressure with sneezing, noseblowing, coughing, or straining. This is followed by the abrupt onset of vertigo.

Patients with *benign positional paroxysmal vertigo* (BPPV) have episodes of vertigo that are precipitated by changes in position such as turning over in bed or looking upward. The attacks are brief, usually lasting seconds to minutes, and symptoms typically begin after a few seconds' latency following the change in position. Attacks occur most frequently when reclining in bed at night on upon awakening in the morning. There may be associated severe nausea and vomiting. Attacks may occur in clusters, with patients asymptomatic for months or years in between.

BPPV results from freely moving crystals of calcium carbonate within one of the semicircular canals. When the head is stationary, these crystals settle in the most dependent part of the canal (usually posterior). With head movements, these crystals move more slowly than the endolymph within which they lie, and their inertia once the head comes to rest causes ongoing stimulation of the hair cells that results in the illusion of movement (vertigo). Diagnosis is established by demonstrating the characteristic downbeating and torsional nystagmus with the Dix-Hallpike test (Fig. 7–1). A positioning (Epley) maneuver (Fig. 7–1) can be used to remove the crystals from the posterior semicircular canal.

◆ KEY POINTS ◆

1. Vertigo is a hallucination of movement that results from acute unilateral vestibular dysfunction.

2. Tinnitus and hearing loss accompany peripheral vertigo; diplopia, dysarthria, or other symptoms of brainstem dysfunction indicate a central cause.

3. Isolated vertigo is almost never caused by brainstem ischemia.

4. Recurrent episodes of vertigo lasting seconds to minutes that are triggered by a change in head position are typical of benign positional paroxysmal vertigo.

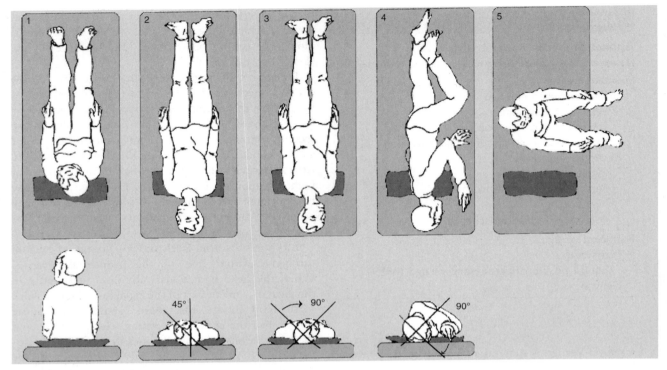

Figure 7–1 The Dix-Hallpike maneuver is illustrated in the first two frames of the figure. The patient's head is rotated 45° to one side and then extended 30° over the edge of the bed. The examiner looks for a rotatory and down-beating nystagmus. The Epley positioning maneuver begins with the positioning used for the Dix-Hallpike maneuver and continues with a series of other positions as illustrated.

SYNCOPE

Syncope is a transient loss of consciousness and postural tone that results from brain hypoperfusion. Prior to losing consciousness, patients often report lightheadedness and a variety of visual symptoms (blurred or tunnel vision, graying or blacking out). The term *presyncope* is used when patients experience this prodrome of symptoms but do not subsequently lose consciousness. Syncope is most commonly a manifestation of hypotension due to cardiac disease, low intravascular volume, or excessive vasodilation. There are essentially two neurologic varieties of syncope, and both involve some dysfunction of the autonomic nervous system. The more common is neurogenic syncope, in which acute hypotension results from transient failure of autonomic cardiovascular control. Less commonly, syncope may result from orthostatic hypotension due to persistent autonomic failure.

Neurogenic syncope is an acute hemodynamic reaction produced by a sudden change in the activity of the autonomic nervous system. Its pathophysiology involves a reflex that is triggered by excessive afferent discharges from arterial (including the heart and great vessels) or visceral mechanoreceptors. Afferent impulses via the vagus nerve lead to cardio-inhibition and vasodepression that result in hypotension and bradycardia. Different terms are used to describe this reflex depending on the trigger (Table 7–2).

Orthostatic hypotension may result from intravascular volume depletion (e.g., dehydration or Addison's disease) or from an inability to activate efferent sympathetic fibers appropriately upon assumption of the upright posture. The underlying pathology is either

TABLE 7–2

Reflex Syncope

Type of Syncope	Pathophysiologic Trigger
Micturition syncope	Rapid emptying of a distended bladder
Carotid sinus hypersensitivity	Compression of the carotid sinus
Neurocardiogenic syncope	Vigorous contraction of an underfilled ventricle
Vasovagal syncope	Strong emotions or acute pain

primary or secondary autonomic failure (e.g., due to diabetic autonomic neuropathy), but the hallmark of both is the failure to release noradrenaline upon standing. Patients usually complain of light-headedness and presyncopal symptoms in response to a sudden change in posture or prolonged standing. There may be associated weakness, fatigue, cognitive slowing, headache, neck pain, or buckling of the legs.

In managing patients with symptomatic orthostatic hypotension, it is important to recognize the potential contribution of drugs such as diuretics, antihypertensives, vasodilators, and antidepressants. Raising the head of the bed will reduce nocturnal diuresis, and patients should be advised to move gradually from the supine to standing position. A variety of drugs are available to ameliorate the symptoms of orthostatic hypotension, with midodrine and fludrocortisone being most commonly used.

◆ KEY POINTS ◆

1. Presyncopal symptoms include light-headedness, headache, neck pain, blurring of vision, cognitive slowing, and buckling of the knees.

2. Syncope results from cerebral hypoperfusion.

3. Neurogenic syncope results from inappropriate activation of a cardio-inhibitory and vasodepressor reflex that may be triggered by micturition, deglutition, carotid sinus compression, sudden underfilling of the ventricle, or heightened vagal tone.

4. Neurogenic orthostatic hypotension results from dysfunction of the autonomic nervous system.

8

Ataxia and Gait Disorders

Ataxia is a term derived from Greek meaning "irregularity" or "disorderliness," and is a general term used to describe the manifestations of diseases of the cerebellum or its connections. It is important, however, to recognize that not all ataxia is cerebellar in origin. For example, the de-afferentation that results from loss of position sense also results in an ataxia. Hence, it is appropriate to distinguish cerebellar ataxia from sensory ataxia.

The cerebellum controls the force, direction, range, rate, and rhythm of movements; a disturbance of these elements results in the signs and symptoms characteristic of cerebellar disease (Table 8–1). Ataxia is not the only process that may underlie a gait disorder, and these other causes are therefore described separately.

ATAXIA

Diagnostic Approach

The spectrum or disorders characterized by prominent ataxia is diverse. A limited differential diagnosis can often be generated by considering the acuity with which symptoms begin and whether the disorder is temporary, episodic, or progressive. It is also helpful to consider the age of onset, the presence of a family history, and the mode of inheritance. A classification based on this approach is outlined in Table 8–2. The details of a few of these disorders are specified below. Associated symptoms and signs may also provide useful diagnostic information; some of these are summarized in Table 8–3. Finally, at a clinical level, a distinction can often be made between lesions of the vermis and cerebellar hemispheres. Vermal lesions typically produce prominent truncal and gait ataxia. Hemispheric lesions, however, typically manifest with ipsilateral limb ataxia.

Cerebellar Hemorrhage or Infarction

Cerebellar hemorrhage or infarction typically presents with the abrupt onset of vertigo, vomiting, and an inability to walk. Level of arousal may be depressed if there is compression of the fourth ventricle with hydrocephalus or if there is pressure on the brainstem. Cerebellar stroke should be considered a medical emergency because neurosurgical intervention may be required for decompression if there is brainstem compression or risk of herniation.

Alcoholic Cerebellar Degeneration

Alcoholic cerebellar degeneration is a consequence of long-standing alcohol abuse and is usually accompanied by an alcoholic polyneuropathy. It is the most common cause of acquired cerebellar degeneration. The vermis bears the brunt of the damage; the presentation, therefore, is usually with progressive gait and truncal ataxia that evolves over a period of weeks or months. Cessation of drinking and supplementation of nutrition offer the best (although limited) chance of improvement.

TABLE 8–1

Signs and Symptoms of Cerebellar Disease

Dysmetria: Abnormality of the range and force of a movement; manifests as erratic, jerky movements with over- and undershooting the target (hence limb or ocular dysmetria)

Intention tremor: Rhythmic side-to-side oscillations of the limb as it approaches the target

Dysdiadochokinesia: Abnormality of the rate and rhythm of a movement demonstrated by asking the patient to perform a rapid alternating movement

Gait ataxia: Broad-based and unsteady, with an inability to walk in a straight line and a tendency to lurch from side to side

Truncal ataxia: Impaired control of truncal posture; when severe, unable even to sit unsupported

Dysarthria: Slow scanning and monotonous speech

Nystagmus

TABLE 8–2

Classification of the Ataxias

Acute or subacute onset with resolution or episodic course
 Postinfectious and infectious cerebellitis
 Cerebellar hemorrhage or infarction
 Drugs (e.g., phenytoin, barbiturates, antineoplastic agents)
 Multiple sclerosis
 Hydrocephalus*
 Posterior fossa mass*
 Foramen magnum compression*
 Dominantly inherited episodic ataxias
 Childhood metabolic disorders (e.g., aminoacidurias, disorders of pyruvate and lactate metabolism)
Acute or subacute onset with progressive course
 Paraneoplastic cerebellar degeneration
 Alcoholic or nutritional cerebellar degeneration
Chronic onset and progressive course
 Autosomal dominant spinocerebellar degenerations
 Autosomal recessive cerebellar degenerative disorders
 Infectious (e.g., Creutzfeldt-Jakob disease)
 Vitamin E deficiency
 Hypothyroidism
 Childhood metabolic disorders (e.g., mitochondrial encephalomyelopathies, Wilson's disease, ataxia-telangiectasia)

*May also cause insidious onset and chronically progressive ataxia.

TABLE 8–3

Associated Symptoms and Signs in Cerebellar Ataxia

Associated Symptom or Sign	Diagnostic Possibilities
Vomiting	Cerebellar stroke, posterior fossa mass
Fever	Viral cerebellitis, infection, or abscess
Malnutrition	Alcoholic cerebellar degeneration or vitamin E deficiency
Depressed consciousness	Cerebellar stroke, childhood metabolic disorders
Dementia	Creutzfeldt-Jacob disease, inherited spinocerebellar ataxia
Optic neuritis or atrophy	Multiple sclerosis
Ophthalmoplegia	Wernicke's encephalopathy, Miller-Fisher syndrome, multiple sclerosis, cerebellar stroke, posterior fossa mass
Extrapyramidal signs	Wilson's disease, Creutzfeldt-Jacob disease, olivopontocerebellar atrophy
Hyporeflexia or areflexia	Miller-Fisher syndrome, Friedreich's ataxia, alcoholic cerebellar degeneration, hypothyroidism
Downbeat nystagmus	Foramen magnum lesion, posterior fossa mass

Postinfectious Cerebellitis

Postinfectious cerebellitis typically affects children between the ages of 2 and 7 and usually follows a varicella or viral infection. Children present with acute onset of limb and gait ataxia as well as dysarthria. Severity ranges from mild unsteadiness to complete inability to walk. The diagnosis is one of exclusion; this usually requires a careful search for underlying drug intoxication as well as a mass lesion in the posterior fossa. The illness lasts a few weeks, and recovery is usually complete.

Paraneoplastic Cerebellar Degeneration

Paraneoplastic cerebellar degeneration (PCD) typically presents with acute or subacute onset of a pancerebellar syndrome with truncal, gait, and limb ataxia; dysarthria; and disturbances of ocular motility (ocular dysmetria, nystagmus). The disease usually evolves to its maximal extent over a period of weeks and then stabilizes, leaving the patient with profound disability. PCD is typically associated with an underlying gynecologic or small cell lung cancer and may become manifest prior to diagnosis of the tumor. Magnetic resonance imaging (MRI) is usually normal. Cerebrospinal fluid may reveal elevated protein or a lymphocytic pleocytosis, but is frequently normal. A variety of autoantibodies (e.g., anti-Yo, anti-Hu) have been described in this condition.

Friedreich's Ataxia

Friedreich's ataxia is an autosomal recessive disorder characterized by progressive ataxia that usually affects the arms more than the legs, as well as by severe dysarthria. Onset is usually in childhood. Classic associated findings are loss of reflexes, spasticity and extensor plantar responses, and impaired vibration and position sense.

Inherited Episodic Ataxia

The episodic ataxia (EA) syndromes are characterized by brief episodes of ataxia, vertigo, nausea, and vomiting. EA-1 is caused by mutations in a voltage-gated potassium channel. Episodes are brief, and there is associated inter-attack skeletal muscle myokymia. EA-2 is caused by mutations in the pore-forming α_1 subunit of the P/Q-type voltage-gated calcium channel. Attacks are longer, lasting several minutes; there is interictal nystagmus; and a progressive irreversible ataxia may develop late in the disease.

Autosomal Dominant Spinocerebellar Degenerations

The clinical diagnosis is based on the occurrence of cerebellar ataxia with or without additional neurologic signs and a family history consistent with autosomal dominant inheritance. The typical presentation is the insidious onset of progressive impairment of gait and dysarthria in young adult life. Associated neurologic abnormalities (e.g., oculomotor, pyramidal, or extrapyramidal signs) may suggest the underlying genotype. Mild to moderate cognitive decline is a late feature in most of the spinocerebellar ataxias (SCAs). All SCAs for which the genetic defect has been identified have been shown to be caused by trinucleotide (CAG) expansions. SCA6 is allelic to EA-2, with the mutated gene being the pore-forming α_1 subunit of the P/Q-type voltage-gated calcium channel. The normal function of the other SCA genes is presently unknown.

Miller-Fisher Syndrome

The Miller-Fisher syndrome is a disorder characterized by the triad of ataxia, areflexia, and ophthalmoplegia. It is thought to be a variant of the Guillain-Barré syndrome and, as such, is most likely mediated by a postinfectious immune process. IgG anti-GQ_{1b} antibodies are detectable in the serum of over 90% of patients with this syndrome. It is usually a self-limiting disorder with a relatively good prognosis for full recovery.

◆ KEY POINTS ◆

1. Sudden onset of cerebellar ataxia with associated vomiting and depressed level of consciousness suggests a cerebellar stroke.

2. Alcoholic cerebellar degeneration typically affects the vermis and manifests with gait and truncal ataxia.

3. Postinfectious cerebellitis is a common cause of ataxia in children.

4. Paraneoplastic cerebellar degeneration is a pancerebellar syndrome and is most often associated with small cell lung cancer or a gynecologic malignancy.

5. The inherited episodic ataxias are caused by mutations in calcium and potassium channel genes.

6. The autosomal dominant SCAs are a group of degenerative disorders caused by trinucleotide expansions.

OTHER GAIT DISORDERS

Abnormalities of gait are common and frequently multifactorial. Not all gait disorders are the result of disease of the nervous system. For example, local mechanical factors such as pain and arthritis may impair ambulation. These factors will not be discussed further here.

Clues to the etiology of the gait disorder may be derived from the presence of other neurologic abnormalities, such as weakness, spasticity, rigidity, bradykinesia, ataxia, or frontal lobe dysfunction. Sometimes, however, an abnormal gait is sufficiently characteristic to permit identification of the underlying disorder based solely on the features of the gait. The following sections are devoted to descriptions of the different types of gait disorders. The differential diagnosis of each type of gait is presented in Table 8–4.

Hemiplegic Gait

The affected leg is stiff and does not flex at the hip, knee, or ankle. The leg is circumducted, with a tendency to scrape the floor with the toes. The arm is held in flexion and adduction and does not swing freely. The spastic (paraparetic) gait is essentially that of a bilateral hemiplegia. The adductor tone is increased, and the legs tend to cross during walking (scissoring gait).

Akinetic-Rigid Gait

Posture is stooped, with flexion of the shoulders, neck, and trunk. Gait is narrow-based, slow, and shuffling with small steps and reduced arm swing. Instead the arms are carried flexed and slightly ahead of the body. There is often difficulty with gait initiation. Postural reflexes are impaired, and the patient may take a series of rapid small steps (festination) forward (propulsion) or backward (retropulsion) in an effort to preserve equilibrium. The foregoing description is typical of patients with idiopathic Parkinson's disease, but may also be seen in other extrapyramidal disorders. One difference in progressive supranuclear palsy is that posture tends toward extension rather than flexion.

Frontal Gait

Posture is flexed and the feet may be slightly apart. Gait initiation is impaired, and the word "magnetic" is used to describe the difficulty in lifting the feet off the ground. The patient advances with small, shuffling, and

TABLE 8–4

Etiology of Various Abnormal Gaits

Gait Disorder	Anatomical Location	Pathology
Hemiplegic	Brainstem, cerebral hemisphere	Stroke, tumor, trauma
Paraplegic	Spinal cord	Demyelination (e.g., multiple sclerosis), transverse myelitis, compressive myelopathy
	Bihemispheral	Diffuse anoxic injury
Akinetic-rigid	Basal ganglia	Parkinson's disease; other parkinsonian syndromes
Frontal	Frontal lobes	Hydrocephalus, tumor, stroke, neurodegenerative disorder
	Subcortical	Binswanger's disease
Waddling	Hip-girdle weakness	Muscular dystrophy, spinal muscular atrophy, acquired proximal myopathy
Slapping	Large-fiber neuropathy	Vitamin B_{12} deficiency
	Dorsal columns	Tabes dorsalis

hesitant steps. With increasing severity, the patient may make abortive stepping movements in one place without the ability to move forward.

Waddling Gait

A waddling gait is characteristic of hip-girdle weakness. During normal walking, the hip abductors contract to fix the weight-bearing leg and thus allow the opposite leg to rise and the trunk to tilt toward the fixed leg. Weakness of the abductors and consequent failure to stabilize the weight-bearing hip cause the pelvis and trunk to tilt toward the opposite side during walking.

Sensory Ataxia

Loss of proprioceptive input from the feet impairs the ability of the patient to determine his position in space. Gait, therefore, becomes cautious. It is wide-based, and steps are slow. Contact with the ground is made by the heel, and the forefoot then strikes the floor with a slapping sound (hence *slapping gait*). Walking on uneven surfaces or in the dark is particularly difficult.

Psychogenic Gait

There is no single typical character to this gait. Instead, a range of abnormalities may be seen. With psychogenic leg weakness, for example, the patient tends to drag the leg behind or push it ahead of her. The circumduction

characteristic of the genuine hemiplegic gait is absent. Another feature is that the patient may adopt extreme postures and lurch wildly in all directions but without falling, thus demonstrating good strength and more than adequate postural reflexes. The term *astasia-abasia* is used to describe this sort of acrobatic psychogenic gait.

◆ **KEY POINTS** ◆

1. Hemiplegic gait suggests hemispheral dysfunction, most often stroke.

2. Paraplegic gait typically suggests spinal cord disease.

3. Akinetic-rigid gait is a feature of parkinsonian syndromes.

4. Frontal gait suggests hydrocephalus (including normal pressure hydrocephalus), neurodegenerative process, or bifrontal or diffuse subcortical disease.

5. Waddling gait suggests proximal muscle (hip-girdle) weakness.

6. Slapping gait indicates large-fiber sensory or dorsal column dysfunction.

9

Urinary and Sexual Dysfunction

Urinary bladder dysfunction is associated with a wide variety of neurologic diseases. Some common conditions are stroke, dementia, Parkinson's disease, multiple sclerosis, and diabetes. A clinical understanding of how these neurologic diseases cause incontinence is important in both diagnosis and management.

ANATOMY AND PHYSIOLOGY OF CONTINENCE

Micturition (voiding) is controlled by neural circuits in the brain and spinal cord that coordinate the activity of visceral smooth muscle in the urinary bladder and urethra with the activity of striated muscle in the external urethral sphincter. These circuits act as on-off switches to shift the lower urinary tract between two modes of operation: storage (sympathetic) and elimination (parasympathetic) (Fig. 9–1).

The different neuroanatomic connections important for bladder control have been defined as "circuits" by Bradley. The first circuit connects the dorsomedial frontal lobe to the medial (M) region in the pons, providing the volitional control of micturition. The second circuit, or spino-bulbo-spinal circuit, is a reflex arc that starts in the urinary bladder and projects to the M region of the pons, with outflow connections to the parasympathetic sacral spinal motor nuclei. The third circuit is a spinal segmental reflex arc with afferent fibers from the detrusor muscle to the pudendal nucleus and

efferent fibers to the striated sphincter muscles (see Fig. 9–1).

M-region stimulation produces a decrease in urethral pressure, followed by a rise in detrusor muscle pressure and voiding. The M region projects to the intermediolateral columns of the sacral cord. The lateral (L) region is at the same level of the pons; its stimulation produces a powerful contraction of the urethral sphincter (storage). Damage at the level of the pontine micturition center will produce a loss of inhibitory control over spinal reflexes. As the bladder becomes distended, the micturition reflex is automatically activated without the patient's awareness or control, and detrusor hyperreflexia and incontinence occur.

Clinical Evaluation

The first objective in the evaluation of bladder incontinence is to determine if the problem is neurogenic or not. A detailed history is essential. Information about initiation; voiding problems such as frequency, stream characteristics, volume of urine, fullness, and urgency; effects of posture, cough, Valsalva maneuver, and medications; and associated bowel and sexual dysfunctions is important.

Thorough physical and neurologic examinations are necessary. The examiner seeks signs of frontal lobe dysfunction, parkinsonian features, sensory level, myelopathy, and so forth. Laboratory evaluation includes basic urinalysis to rule out infection. Urodynamic studies can clarify the characteristics of the incontinence, determine

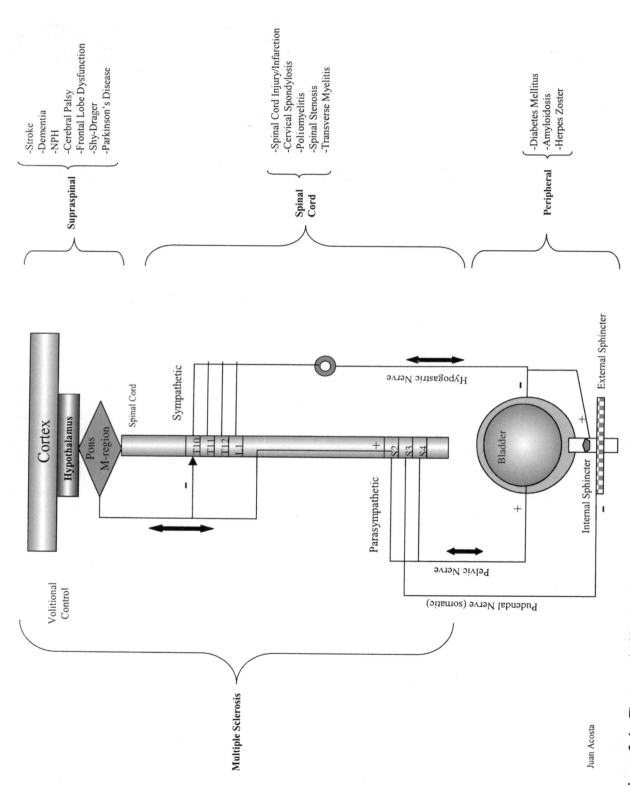

Figure 9–1   The control of bladder function.

Suprapinal

-Stroke
-Dementia
-NPH
-Cerebral Palsy
-Frontal Lobe Dysfunction
-Shy-Drager
-Parkinson's Disease

Spinal Cord

-Spinal Cord Injury/Infarction
-Cervical Spondylosis
-Poliomyelitis
-Spinal Stenosis
-Transverse Myelitis

Peripheral

-Diabetes Mellitus
-Amyloidosis
-Herpes Zoster

Cortex
Hypothalamus
Pons
M-region
Spinal Cord

Sympathetic

T10
T11
T12
L1

Parasympathetic

S2
S3
S4

Hypogastric Nerve
Pelvic Nerve
Pudendal Nerve (somatic)

Bladder
Internal Sphincter
External Sphincter

Volitional Control

Multiple Sclerosis

Juan Acosta

the underlying neurologic abnormality, categorize the vesicourethral dysfunction, and provide a basis for appropriate therapy. Measurement of the postvoid residual (PVR) by bladder ultrasound or catheterization is important in the characterization of bladder dysfunction. The PVR represents the residual volume in the bladder after voiding. A normal PVR is less than 50 mL.

Other urodynamic studies include the following:

- *Cystometry:* Provides information about bladder compliance, capacity, and volume at first sensation and at urge to void; voiding pressure; and the presence of uninhibited detrusor contractions
- *Cystourethroscopy:* Assesses the integrity of the lower urinary system, and identifies important urethral and bladder lesions
- *Retrograde urethrography*
- *Neurophysiologic studies:* Includes sphincter and pelvic floor electromyography (EMG)

Urodynamic findings in various types of neurogenic bladder dysfunction are listed in Table 9–1.

◆ **KEY POINTS** ◆

1. The M region is the site of activation of micturition in the pons.

2. History and a complete neurologic exam are important in the evaluation of bladder incontinence.

3. PVR should be less than 50 mL. Increased PVR implies poor bladder emptying. Sphincter dyssynergia and atonic bladder are common neurogenic causes of elevated PVR.

CLASSIFICATION OF INCONTINENCE

Based on the patient symptoms, the following types of incontinence are recognized.

Urge incontinence is an involuntary loss of urine associated with a strong desire to void (urgency), usually associated with detrusor instability (DI). When the DI is the result of a neurologic problem, the term *detrusor hyperreflexia* (DH) is used; its clinical expression is a spastic bladder. DH is common in patients with strokes, suprasacral spinal cord lesions, and multiple sclerosis. It is usually accompanied by detrusor-sphincter dyssynergia (DSD), which is inappropriate contraction of the external sphincter with detrusor contraction. This can result in urinary retention, vesicourethral reflux, and subsequent renal damage.

Stress incontinence is an involuntary loss of urine during coughing, sneezing, laughing, or other physical activities that increase intra-abdominal pressure (in the absence of detrusor contraction or an overdistended bladder). This is common in multiparous women who have cystoceles or weakness of muscles of the pelvic floor. Other causes include urethral hypermobility; significant displacement of the urethra and bladder neck; and intrinsic urethral sphincter deficiency due to congenital weakness in patients with myelomeningocele or epispadias or who have had prostatectomy, trauma, or radiation.

Mixed incontinence is a combination of urge and stress incontinence.

Overflow incontinence is an involuntary loss of urine associated with overdistention of the bladder. Patients report constant dribbling, or urge or stress incontinence symptoms. The resultant atonic bladder can be produced by an underactive or acontractile detrusor (due to drugs, diabetic neuropathy, lower spinal cord injury, or

---

TABLE 9–1

Urodynamic Findings in Neurogenic Bladder

Type	Capacity	Compliance	Others
Spastic bladder	Decreased	Reduced	Uninhibited detrusor contractions
Atonic bladder	Increased	Increased	Low voiding pressure and flow rate

radical pelvic surgery that interrupts innervation of the detrusor muscle). Bladder outlet and urethral obstruction can also cause overdistention and overflow.

◆　KEY POINTS　◆

1. Spastic bladder implies an upper motor neuron problem due to lesions involving the frontal lobes, pons, or suprasacral spinal cord. Symptoms are incontinence with urgency. Urodynamics show decreased capacity and reduced compliance.

2. Atonic bladder implies a lower motor neuron lesion at the level of the conus medullaris, cauda equina, or sacral plexus, or peripheral nerve dysfunction. It is characterized by overflow incontinence and increased capacity and compliance.

3. Sphincter dyssynergia produces an increased PVR with fluctuating voiding pressures and intermittent flow rate.

4. A small PVR is good; a large PVR with spastic or atonic bladder is not. It can cause increased intrabladder pressure with deleterious effect on the ureters and kidneys.

INCONTINENCE IN THE NEUROLOGIC PATIENT

The evaluation of urinary incontinence in the neurologic patient requires a detailed physical and neurologic exam in an attempt to define the level of the lesion. Lesions can be localized to the following levels: supraspinal, spinal, peripheral, and mixed.

Supraspinal Diseases

Supraspinal diseases usually result in a hyperreflexic bladder, causing urge incontinence, a small bladder capacity, and small PVR, with no deleterious effects on the upper urinary tract because voiding is unobstructed.

Cerebrovascular Disease

Large strokes (particularly frontal or pontine) produce an upper motor neuron bladder (hyperreflexic and small with urgency and frequency). Urinary incontinence after stroke is common and is associated with overall poor functional outcome.

Parkinson's Disease

Voiding dysfunction occurs in 40% to 70% of patients with Parkinson's disease. Detrusor hyperreflexia is the most common finding. Pseudodyssynergia occurs as a consequence of sphincter bradykinesia. Urologic causes such as benign prostatic hypertrophy are frequently associated.

Spinal Cord Diseases

Spinal cord diseases represent the most common cause of neurogenic bladder dysfunction. In a clinical study, 74% of patients with neurogenic bladder dysfunction had some form of spinal cord disease.

Following disconnection from the pons, the sphincter tends to contract when the detrusor is contracting (dyssynergia). New reflexes emerge to drive bladder emptying and cause detrusor hyperreflexia. During spinal shock the bladder is acontractile, but gradually over weeks reflex detrusor contractions develop in response to low filling volumes.

Spinal Cord Injury

Spinal cord injury produces detrusor hyperreflexia, loss of compliance, and detrusor-sphincter dyssynergia.

Multiple Sclerosis

About 75% of patients with multiple sclerosis (MS) have bladder dysfunction. About 65% complain of irritative symptoms, 25% of obstructive symptoms, and 10% of mixed symptoms. Detrusor hyperreflexia occurs in 50% to 90% of patients, among whom 50% also have detrusor-sphincter dyssynergia.

Peripheral Nerve Diseases

Because of its extensive autonomic innervation, bladder dysfunction is most often seen in those generalized polyneuropathies involving small nerve fibers. Urodynamic studies show impaired detrusor contractility, decreased bladder sensation, decreased flow rate, and increased PVR. A classic example is diabetic cystopathy, in which a progressive loss of bladder sensation and impairment of bladder emptying eventually results in chronic low-pressure urinary retention. The situation is similar in other types of neuropathies such as amyloidosis, immune-mediated polyneuropathies (25% of Guillain-Barré patients have bladder symptoms), and inherited neuropathies. Injury to pelvic nerves can produce similar symptoms (e.g., local radiation or surgery).

◆ **KEY POINTS** ◆

1. Stroke and spinal cord disease usually produce an upper motor neuron bladder or spastic bladder with or without sphincter dyssynergia.

2. Small-fiber neuropathies can produce a neurogenic atonic bladder with high PVR.

TREATMENT OF URINARY INCONTINENCE

Therapy for a neurogenic bladder includes pharmacologic and nonpharmacologic approaches. Some of the behavioral techniques that may help with the treatment of this condition include toileting assistance, bladder retraining, and pelvic muscle rehabilitation.

Pharmacologic agents are available to treat bladder dysfunction. The choice of therapy is based on an understanding of the underlying mechanism of the dysfunction and therefore the site of the neural injury.

Table 9–2 summarizes treatments for urinary incontinence.

◆ **KEY POINTS** ◆

1. Therapy of urinary incontinence is individualized and often requires adjustments.

2. The main management goals are preservation of upper urinary tract function and improvement of the patient's urinary symptoms that impair quality of life.

ERECTILE DYSFUNCTION

The sexual response cycle of excitement, plateau, orgasm, and resolution requires the integrated and coordinated activity of the somatic and autonomic nervous systems innervating the reproductive system. Erectile dysfunction (ED) is defined as the persistent inability to attain or maintain penile erection sufficient for sexual intercourse.

An estimated 10 to 20 million American men have some degree of ED. Biologic or organic causes are demonstrated in up to 80% of cases, though psychiatric or psychogenic factors are important.

Anatomy and Physiology

The pudendal nerve carries both the motor and sensory fibers that innervate the penis and clitoris. The parasympathetic nerves are located in the sacral cord (S2 through S4) and participate in erection. The sympathetic nerves arise from cells in the T11 to T12 level of the spinal cord through the hypogastric plexus and are important in ejaculation.

Local mediators such as nitric oxide and guanosine monophosphate (cGMP) are primarily released by parasympathetic activity contributing to sustained erection.

Causes of Sexual Dysfunction

The etiology of sexual dysfunction can be multifactorial. Neurogenic causes include neuropathy, myelopathy, cauda equina lesions, and central nervous system dysfunction. Other causes include vascular disease, pelvic trauma, and endocrine disorders such as hypothyroidism, hypogonadism, and hyperprolactinemia. Chronic illness, psychogenic illness, and drugs (i.e., antihypertensives, anticholinergics, antidepressants, sedatives, and narcotics) are frequent causes. Metabolic and toxic disorders such as alcohol abuse, liver disease, and renal failure are also common causes.

Clinical Evaluation

The evaluation of a patient with ED includes a complete history and physical exam. Neurologic examination may provide evidence of cerebral, spinal cord, or peripheral nerve dysfunction. Laboratory evaluation includes an endocrine panel with levels of prolactin, testosterone, and gonadotropins. Sleep studies can be helpful (erection usually occurs with each REM episode). EMG and somatosensory evoked potentials can help in cases of myelopathy or peripheral nerve disease. Vascular studies evaluate the response of the penis to the injection of vasoactive agents such as papaverine.

Management of Erectile Dysfunction

The management of ED requires the recognition of the etiology and the treatment of the underlying disease.

TABLE 9–2

Treatment of Urinary Incontinence

Type	Therapy	Notes

Urge incontinence (spastic bladder)	1. Anticholinergic agents
	  a. Tolterodine (Detrol), 2 mg bid
	  b. Oxybutynin (Ditropan), 2.5–5.0 mg po tid/qid
	  c. Propantheline, 7.5–30.0 mg tid/qid
	2. Tricyclic antidepressants
	  a. Imipramine, 25 mg po tid/qid
	3. Desmopressin (DDAVP) spray or tablets
		Tolterodine is tolerated better than oxybutynin. Most frequent side effect: dry mouth. Others include headache, dyspepsia, dizziness, and urinary tract infections.
		
		Desmopressin is used to treat diabetes insipidus; however, it produces a significant reduction in voiding frequency in the 6 hours following treatment. Use only *once* a day.

	4. Intravesical capsaicin	Intravesical capsaicin is used for intractable detrusor hyperreflexia. It has a neurotoxic effect on the afferent C fibers that drive volume-determined reflex detrusor contractions. Lessening of urgency and frequency may last up to 6 months.

Stress incontinence	1. Alpha-adrenergic agonist drugs
	  a. Phenylpropanolamine, 25–100 mg bid
	  b. Pseudoephedrine, 15–30 mg tid
	2. Estrogen therapy, oral or vaginal
		Alpha-adrenergic agonist drugs stimulate smooth muscle alpha-adrenergic receptors.
		
		Estrogen therapy is adjunctive for postmenopausal women with stress or mixed incontinence.

Atonic bladder with overflow incontinence	1. Credé's maneuver or Valsalva maneuver to empty the bladder. 2. Intermittent self-catheterization is perhaps the mainstay of long-term treatment. 3. Pharmacotherapy is usually not an effective treatment modality. The cholinergic agent bethanecol (25–50 mg tid/qid) is used.	Bethanechol stimulates cholinergic receptors, increasing detrusor muscle tone. Side effects include bronchospasm, diarrhea, abdominal pain, and flushing.
Detrusor dyssynergia	1. Intermittent catheterization 2. Suprapubic catheterization. 3. Sacral nerve stimulation	

Endocrine, metabolic, vascular, and psychogenic etiologies must be treated when present. If drugs are responsible, changes in medication may be beneficial. Discussion of available medical and surgical treatments is beyond the focus of this chapter.

Pharmacologic therapy of ED includes sildenafil (Viagra) used in doses of 25 to 100 mg, 30 to 60 minutes before intercourse (side effects include facial flushing and headache), intraurethral suppositories and intracavernosal injections of alprostadil (Caverject).

◆ KEY POINTS ◆

1. ED affects an estimated 10 to 20 million Americans.

2. ED is often multifactorial. Many neurogenic diseases can produce ED, including strokes, multiple sclerosis, and diabetes.

3. Medical and surgical therapies are available. Sildenafil (Viagra) is a new oral medication with good results in many patients.

10

Headache and Facial Pain

Headache is one of the most common symptoms encountered by physicians. Approximately 70% to 80% of the population has headaches at some time, and 50% have headaches at least once per month. The challenge of treating patients with headache lies not only in treatment but also in determining when headache represents a symptom of more serious disease. Therefore, the approach to the patient with headache entails understanding the pathophysiology of head pain, performing a complete history and physical exam, generating a differential diagnosis, and pursuing treatment options.

PATHOPHYSIOLOGY

Headache is caused by a disturbance or irritation of the pain-sensitive structures in the head. Within the cranium, pain-sensitive structures include blood vessels, meninges, and cranial nerves V, IX, and X. Outside the cranium, the pain-sensitive structures are the periosteum of the skull, muscles, nerves, arteries and veins, subcutaneous tissues, eyes, ears, sinuses, and mucous membranes. Of note, the brain parenchyma itself and bones are insensitive to pain. Tumors or hydrocephalus cause pain by producing enough mass effect to result in stretching of pain-sensitive structures such as the meninges or blood vessels.

Irritation or damage to the pain-sensitive structures results in nociceptive information being relayed to the brain via cranial nerve V (trigeminal) or by the upper cervical roots. In addition to the dermatomal innervation of the trigeminal nerve (Fig. 10–1), the anterior and middle cranial fossas are innervated by cranial nerve V, especially V_1, while the upper cervical roots innervate structures in the posterior fossa. Thus, painful stimulation of structures in the anterior or middle fossa is often referred to the eye or front or side of the head, whereas painful stimulation of structures in the posterior fossa results in pain that is referred to the back of the head and upper part of the neck.

◆ **KEY POINTS** ◆

1. Pain-sensitive structures inside the skull include blood vessels, meninges, and cranial nerves V, IX, and X.
2. Cranial nerve V relays nociceptive information from the pain-sensitive structures inside the skull to the brain.

HISTORY AND PHYSICAL EXAM

Generally, headaches should be classified into three major categories:

1. Primary headaches that represent the common headache syndromes such as migraine, cluster, and

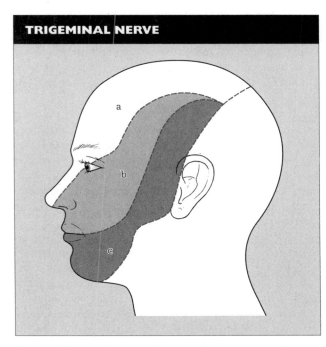

TRIGEMINAL NERVE

Figure 10–1   Sensory division of the trigeminal nerve (cranial nerve V): (a) ophthalmic division, or V₁; (b) maxillary division, or V₂; (c) mandibular division, or V₃. (Reproduced with permission from Ginsberg, L. Lecture notes on neurology. Malden, MA: Blackwell Science, 1999:32.)

tension headaches. These headaches should not be associated with an underlying structural cause.

2. Headaches related to serious neurologic diseases such as brain tumor, meningitis, and aneurysm.

3. Headaches or pain from structures in the skull and face such as the eyes, sinuses, and mouth.

The history and physical exam should be aimed at differentiating the above possibilities. Onset and frequency aid in the diagnosis of chronic headache. A new sudden severe headache that has never occurred before may be a symptom of aneurysm rupture causing subarachnoid hemorrhage. A progressively worsening headache over the last month or so may indicate a slowly expanding tumor, whereas a frequent headache that has been present for twenty years usually implies a more benign etiology.

Location of pain, such as tenderness over the sinuses (sinusitis) or the temporomandibular joint can help dif-

ferentiate these conditions from a primary headache disorder. Migraine and cluster headaches are often unilateral, whereas tension headaches are usually bilateral. Prodromal symptoms such as scintillating scotoma can be associated with classic migraine headaches or postictal headaches in patients with a seizure disorder. Precipitating factors are also an important guide to identifying the etiology of headache. Alcohol is often a trigger for cluster headache, whereas nitrite-containing foods (hot dogs, salami, and other preserved meats) and cheeses containing tyramine can trigger migraine headaches.

Description of pain is also useful in characterizing headache or facial pain. Lancinating or shooting pain in a V₂ or V₃ distribution of the trigeminal nerve is characteristic of trigeminal neuralgia (tic douloureux). Unilateral throbbing pain is common in migraine, whereas a dull, bandlike or tightening pain can be associated with tension headache. A sharp, stabbing pain especially behind one eye is common in cluster headaches.

Associated symptoms and neurologic signs are an extremely important aid in the diagnosis of headache and facial pain conditions. Nausea and vomiting can be associated either with migraine headaches or raised intracranial pressure from hydrocephalus or a tumor. Photophobia, phonophobia, or increased frequency of the headache at menstruation can be associated with migraine. Systemic symptoms such as fever can suggest meningitis or a local infection such as a dental abscess as the cause of pain. Unilateral lacrimation or rhinorrhea is associated with cluster headaches.

Warning signs during the history that should alert one to the possibility of a more serious cause of the headache are sudden onset of a new headache or a progressively worsening headache. Headaches associated with a change in level of consciousness can be due to tumor or subarachnoid hemorrhage. Fever, neurologic symptoms or signs, or new headache after the age of 50 should prompt consideration for a serious cause of the headache.

The physical exam should be complete, including registration of vital signs to exclude fever, but particular attention should be focused on the head and neck. Inspection of the entire head should be performed, noting the shape of the head (especially in children who may have hydrocephalus) and identifying signs of trauma. The conjunctiva or iris can appear irritated with primary ocular disorders or with cluster headaches. Auscultation of the carotid arteries may reveal bruits, and auscultation with the bell over the orbits may reveal bruits from an arteriovenous malformation. Palpation can often reveal tight and tender cervical muscles, often found in patients with tension headaches. Tenderness of the temporal arteries in an elderly person may indicate temporal arteritis, while palpation of the temporomandibular joints when the jaw is opened and closed may indicate temporomandibular joint dysfunction. Sinus tenderness during palpation may indicate sinusitis, and tenderness to palpation of the teeth may indicate a dental abscess. Signs of meningeal irritation (see Chapter 21) should be sought especially in patients with fever. Detailed cranial nerve examination should be performed, including funduscopic examination to look for papilledema as a sign of increased intracranial pressure. Partial oculomotor nerve (third cranial nerve) palsy identified by a unilateral dilated pupil can be associated with uncal herniation or an aneurysm of the posterior communicating artery. A unilateral Horner's syndrome can be seen either with cluster headache or carotid artery dissection. Trigger points causing pain in the trigeminal nerve distribution (especially V_2 and V_3) of the face or of the pharynx can suggest trigeminal neuralgia or glossopharyngeal neuralgia, respectively.

PRIMARY HEADACHE DISORDERS

Headaches that do not have an underlying structural cause are called primary headaches. These headaches are diagnosed based on their clinical features, which reinforces the importance of a good history. The main types of primary headaches are migraine, tension-type, and cluster.

Migraine

Migraine headaches can be unilateral or bilateral and pulsing or throbbing in quality. They affect women more commonly than men. Age of onset is typically in the teens or early twenties, and migraines are often associated with nausea and vomiting, photophobia, and phonophobia. Migraine headaches can be associated with an aura, which is a transient focal neurologic symptom that usually precedes the headache and often lasts between 15 minutes and 1 hour.

Migraines with aura are also called classic migraines; migraines without aura are called common migraines. The most common type of aura is visual and can consist of flashing lights or zigzag lines that march across the patient's visual field. Sensory or motor symptoms are also observed. Most auras develop over 5 to 20 minutes, usually in a marching fashion in which the symptoms spread gradually, and rarely last longer than 1 hour. The headache usually follows the aura within 20 to 60 minutes, but some patients have aura only. The headache usually lasts from 4 to 72 hours.

Treatment is aimed at either preventing or aborting an attack. Prevention can be attempted by avoiding triggers such as aged cheese, red wine, and other foods that precipitate an attack. Prophylactic medications such as beta-blockers (propranolol), calcium channel antagonists (verapamil), tricyclic antidepressants (amitriptyline), and some anticonvulsants (valproic acid) can decrease the frequency and severity of attacks.

Abortive therapy is considered in order to stop an acute attack. Simple analgesics such as acetaminophen, aspirin, or prescription-strength nonsteroidal anti-inflammatory drugs (NSAIDs) may be effective if taken early during headache symptoms. Ergot alkaloids and selective serotonin (5-HT_1) agonists (sumatriptan) are effective medications but are contraindicated in patients with uncontrolled hypertension or coronary artery disease because of their vasoconstrictive properties.

Tension-Type Headache

Tension-type headache is a chronic headache that lacks the clinical features of migraine or cluster headache. The underlying pathophysiologic mechanism of the headache is unknown. Muscle spasm may be involved, but controversy exists as to whether the muscle spasm is an epiphenomenon or causal. The pain is usually bilateral and occipital and sometimes described as a tight band around the head. The pain is usually nonthrobbing and affects women somewhat more frequently than men.

There is some thought that tension-type headache is related to migraine and that they are on opposite ends of a clinical continuum. Many of the same medications used in treating migraines are effective for tension-type headaches. In addition to pharmacologic treatment, physical therapy, stress management, biofeedback, and psychotherapy may be beneficial.

Cluster Headaches

Unlike the other primary headache disorders, cluster headaches affect men approximately six times more frequently than women. As the name implies, the headaches usually occur in clusters in which the headaches recur cyclically followed by remission. Headaches usually occur one to three times per day during a cluster that can last up to several months. The remission period can be months to years. The pain typically occurs after work or within several hours of sleep onset and is typically located behind one eye or over the lateral part of the nose. The pain can be extremely severe, and patients commonly have ipsilateral conjunctival injection, lacrimation, nasal congestion, and, less frequently, Horner's syndrome.

Treatment is aimed at avoiding possible precipitants such as alcohol or strenuous exercise during an attack. For prophylaxis, verapamil can be used. Symptomatic treatment of cluster headache is inhalation of pure oxygen, which is over 90% effective. Sumatriptan and dihydroergotamine can also be used.

◆ **KEY POINTS** ◆

1. Primary headaches do not have an underlying structural cause.
2. Table 10–1 summarizes the features of primary headaches.

SECONDARY HEADACHES

As mentioned previously, headache can result from a myriad of underlying etiologies. The following examples are not all-inclusive but illustrate either common neurologic causes of headache or particularly dangerous causes that should be considered in the differential diagnosis.

Subarachnoid Hemorrhage

A nontraumatic subarachnoid hemorrhage is caused by rupture of an aneurysm or bleeding from an arteriovenous malformation. These headaches are sudden and typically severe and oftentimes represent the worst headache of one's life. Loss of consciousness, vomiting, and neck stiffness are common features. Computed tomography (CT) or lumbar puncture looking for evidence of hemorrhage or heme breakdown in the cerebrospinal fluid (CSF) makes the diagnosis. Treatment in the acute setting involves stabilization in an intensive care unit for management of blood pressure for adequate brain perfusion, and monitoring for vasospasm and acute obstructive hydrocephalus caused by the subarachnoid blood. Definitive treatment involves surgical resection or clipping of the aneurysm by a neurosurgeon or coiling by an interventional neuroradiologist.

Temporal Arteritis

Temporal arteritis (giant cell arteritis) is a subacute granulomatous inflammatory condition involving the branches of the external carotid artery, especially the temporal arteries. This disorder occurs almost exclusively in the elderly and is rare in patients younger than 50 years old. It is characterized by headache that can be unilateral or bilateral, particularly over the temporal arteries. Scalp tenderness may be present, and jaw pain during chewing (jaw claudication) may be a clue to the diagnosis. Involvement of the ophthalmic artery can lead to blindness. Thus, the diagnosis must be considered in an elderly patient with a new or worsening

---

TABLE 10–1

Features of Primary Headaches

Primary Headache Type	Male-Female Ratio	Age of Onset	Typical Clinical Features
Migraine Classic Common	F > M	Teen years	Can be unilateral or bilateral, typically throbbing Associated with aura No aura
Tension-type	M = F	Any age	Usually bilateral and occipital or frontal. Pain is typically dull or bandlike
Cluster	M > F	Third decade of life	Pain behind one eye, associated with ipsilateral conjunctival injection, lacrimation, nasal congestion, and occasional Horner's syndrome

headache, especially involving the temporal region, and urgent evaluation must be initiated.

Temporal arteritis is usually associated with an elevated erythrocyte sedimentation rate (ESR) to approximately 100. However, definitive diagnosis is made by temporal artery biopsy demonstrating histologic vasculitis. Multiple biopsies may be required because the vessel can be affected in a patchy manner, and the first site of biopsy may miss the inflamed portion of vessel. Treatment is prednisone in decreasing doses for several months and then continued for the next 1 to 2 years.

Trigeminal Neuralgia

Trigeminal neuralgia (tic douloureux) is a facial pain syndrome in which brief severe electrical shock–like pains occur in the distribution of one of the branches of the trigeminal nerve. The second or third divisions of the trigeminal nerve are most commonly involved. Trigeminal neuralgia is more common in middle-aged and elderly patients. Movement, a cold breeze, or tactile stimulation in a trigger zone on the face can precipitate an attack. The etiology is not completely known but is thought to be due to microvascular compression of the trigeminal nerve. Multiple sclerosis and tumors can cause similar pain episodes and should be ruled out, particularly in younger patients. Carbamazepine is particularly effective in treating trigeminal neuralgia. If ineffective, surgical decompression can be considered.

Idiopathic Intracranial Hypertension (Pseudotumor Cerebri)

Idiopathic intracranial hypertension can affect individuals of any age group but is more common in patients in the second to fourth decades of life. It is more common in women, and there is an association with obesity. In addition to headache, there are often associated visual symptoms that tend to be bilateral and can include fleeting loss of visual acuity, scotoma, or double vision. Neurologic exam is normal except for papilledema that may be present on funduscopic exam. CT or magnetic resonance imaging (MRI) of the head is normal, and lumbar puncture shows elevated pressure that is typically greater than 250 mm of water.

The pathophysiology of idiopathic intracranial hypertension is not known. Treatment usually includes acetazolamide, a carbonic anhydrase inhibitor that inhibits CSF formation. Alternatively, the diuretic, furosemide, or oral steroids can be used. Serial lumbar punctures to reduce the CSF pressure can also be performed. If visual symptoms persist or worsen, a surgeon can perform optic nerve sheath fenestration to decrease papilledema. If treatment is not effective, patients may be left with permanent visual loss.

Post–Lumbar Puncture or Low Pressure Headache

Post–lumbar puncture headache is characterized by headache in an upright position following lumbar puncture. The headache usually starts within 48 hours of the lumbar puncture. The headache is usually relieved when the patient lies down, and typically resolves in several days without specific treatment. If the headache continues, medications, such as intravenous caffeine sodium benzoate, or a blood patch can alleviate the headache. The blood patch is a procedure in which peripheral blood is injected into the epidural space at the site of the lumbar puncture. A clot is formed, sealing the small puncture site in the thecal sac where CSF leakage resulted in traction of pain-sensitive structures in the head.

Other Neurologic Causes

Other neurologic causes of headache are numerous and include brain tumors, increased intracranial pressure from a variety of causes including meningitis, and some types of seizures and strokes. These topics are discussed in more detail in other chapters of this book.

◆ KEY POINTS ◆

1. Sudden onset of severe headache is suspicious for subarachnoid hemorrhage due to aneurysmal rupture.

2. Temporal arteritis occurs in the elderly and requires urgent evaluation because it can cause blindness.

3. Temporal arteritis is often associated with pain over the temporal arteries and an elevated ESR.

Part III
Neurologic
Disorders

Aphasia and Other Disorders of Higher Cortical Function

Disorders of higher cortical function are some of the most interesting in neurology to both physicians and laypersons. Stories of patients who have lost particular aspects of language or who mistake a wife for a hat, for example, continue to intrigue medical students and residents.

It is not hard to understand why this might be: Although primary vision, sensation, and motor control are clearly brain functions that are essential for day-to-day survival, it is the more developed cognitive functions that allow us to carry out the activities that seem *human*. The fact that these functions reside in some fairly discrete areas of the brain and can be quite selectively damaged by lesions in these areas contributes to our fascination with them.

APHASIA

Aphasia refers to any acquired abnormality of language, usually from a focal brain lesion. The problem must be a primary disorder of language; not everyone who cannot communicate properly is aphasic. For example, diffuse problems with consciousness, attention, or initiative may prevent a patient from communicating by oral or written means, but this would not necessarily qualify as aphasia. Likewise, problems with speech, such as dysarthria (slurring) or stuttering, or problems with motor control of the mouth may prevent oral communication, but pronunciation deficits should not be confused with aphasia.

Diagnosis

There are several recognized forms of aphasia (Table 11–1) that are typically caused by lesions in particular brain locations (Fig. 11–1) and which can be distinguished from each other by testing certain aspects of language, such as fluency, comprehension, and repetition (Table 11–2).

A sensitive test for detecting an aphasia of any kind is to test naming, since *anomia* (impaired naming) is a feature of essentially all aphasias. Severely aphasic patients may not be able to name common, or high-frequency, objects (e.g., watch, necktie), while less severely afflicted patients may only have trouble with low-frequency objects or parts (e.g., dial of the watch, lapel). In addition, no aphasic patient writes normally. Screening for aphasia by asking patients to write a paragraph is quite effective.

◆ KEY POINTS ◆

1. Aphasia is an acquired abnormality of language, usually from a focal brain lesion.

2. Other causes of impaired communication, including problems with attention, initiative, or articulation, are not truly aphasias.

3. Problems with naming or writing are features of almost all types of aphasia.

TABLE 11–1

Aphasias

Type	Fluency	Repetition	Comprehension	Commonly Associated Signs	Lesion Location
Broca's	Impaired	Impaired	Relatively preserved	Right hemiparesis (especially face)	Broca's area
Wernicke's	Preserved	Impaired	Impaired	Right upper visual field cut	Wernicke's area
Conduction	Preserved	Impaired	Preserved	—	Arcuate fasciculus
Transcortical motor	Impaired	Preserved	Preserved	Right hemiparesis	Near Broca's area
Transcortical sensory	Preserved	Preserved	Impaired	—	Near Wernicke's area
Global	Impaired	Impaired	Impaired	Severe right hemiparesis	Large left hemisphere lesion
Subcortical	Variable	Preserved	Variable	Hypophonia	Left basal ganglia, thalamus

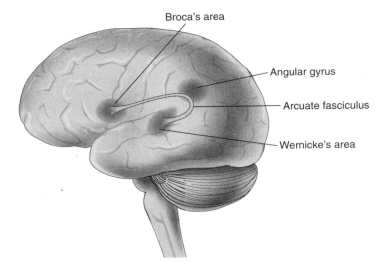

Figure 11–1   Higher cortical centers in the left hemisphere.

Broca's Aphasia

Broca's aphasia is primarily a problem of language production. Speech is nonfluent, meaning that the patient cannot produce a reasonably long string of words. Attempted speech output is punctuated by hesitations and ill-fated attempts at beginnings of words ("tip-of-the-tongue" phenomenon). A Broca's patient's speech may be telegraphic, in that conjunctions, prepositions, and the like may be omitted and only key nouns and verbs strung together (e.g., "want go store"). Patients' speech may include paraphasias (word substitution errors), often of the phonemic type (substitution based

TABLE 11–2

Examination of Language Function

Function	Testing
Fluency	Listen to patient's spontaneous speech to see if words are strung together into phrases. Overused phrases (e.g., "how do you do") do not count.
Repetition	Least challenging: Ask patient to repeat single words.
	Most challenging: Ask patient to repeat complex sentence, such as "no ifs, ands, or buts about it."
Comprehension	Least challenging: Ask patient to follow simple midline commands, such as "close your eyes" or "open your mouth."
	Most challenging: Ask patient to follow multistep appendicular commands that cross the midline, such as "point to the ceiling, then touch your left ear with your right hand."
Naming	Least challenging: Ask patient to name high-frequency objects, like watch or tie.
	Most challenging: Ask patient to name low-frequency objects or parts of objects, like dial of watch or lapel.
Reading	Ask patient to read written material aloud, and to follow written instructions.
Writing	Ask patient to write a spontaneous sentence, or a sentence dictated by the examiner. Simply having the patient write his name does not count, as that is an overlearned task.

on sound, like "spool" for "spoon"). An important feature of Broca's aphasia is that patients are quite aware of and almost invariably frustrated by their language problem. Oddly, overused phrases (e.g., "how do you do"), expletives, and lyrics sung to music may be relatively preserved. Broca's patients cannot repeat phrases said to them. Although the most prominent deficit is with language output, Broca's aphasia patients have subtle deficits of comprehension, particularly for complex grammatical constructions involving prepositions or the passive voice. For example, Broca's patients may not be able to follow a command such as "under the paper put the pen" or understand which animal is dead if "the lion was killed by the tiger."

Classically, Broca's aphasia arises from lesions that include the posterior part of the inferior frontal gyrus in the dominant (usually left) hemisphere, a region known as Broca's area. Most often these are relatively large strokes in the territory of the superior division of the middle cerebral artery (MCA), although tumors, hemorrhages, and other lesions in this area can cause an identical syndrome. Strokes here typically are associated with some weakness of the contralateral side, particularly involving the face and arm.

◆ KEY POINTS ◆

1. Broca's aphasia is a problem of language production.

2. Patients are frustrated and have nonfluent, hesitant, telegraphic speech output with an inability to repeat but relatively preserved comprehension.

3. Broca's aphasia is typically caused by lesions in the posterior inferior frontal lobe (Broca's area).

Wernicke's Aphasia

Although Wernicke's aphasia is often characterized as a problem with language comprehension, it features difficulty with both language output and input. Patients cannot understand what is said to them, and thus may not be able to follow even the simplest commands. Their spontaneous speech is fluent but nonsensical, so they can string words together but the sequence or content may not make sense ("word salad"). Wernicke's patients produce many paraphasias, particularly of the semantic type (substitution based on meaning, like "fork" for "spoon") as well as neologisms (nonexistent words). The cadence and fluency of speech are preserved, but the content is often incomprehensible. One might not be able to recognize that a speaker of a foreign language had a Wernicke's aphasia, because all but the content of language would be intact. Wernicke's aphasia patients cannot repeat. Unlike patients with Broca's aphasia, those with Wernicke's aphasia seem unaware of their deficit initially and can become quite angry or paranoid when it becomes obvious that others have difficulty understanding them.

Classically, Wernicke's aphasia arises from lesions in the posterior part of the superior temporal gyrus in the dominant hemisphere, known as Wernicke's area. Most commonly these are strokes involving the inferior division of the MCA, and a high percentage of them are due to emboli from proximal locations such as the heart or the internal carotid artery. However, other nonvascular lesions in this area can cause an identical syndrome. Lesions causing Wernicke's aphasia may not be accompanied by weakness or sensory loss, but there may be a contralateral homonymous superior quadrantanopia.

◆ KEY POINTS ◆

1. Wernicke's aphasia is a problem with language comprehension that results in difficulties with both language output and input.

2. Patients have fluent but very abnormal speech output ("word salad"), frequent paraphasias and neologisms, and an inability to comprehend or repeat.

3. Wernicke's aphasia is typically caused by lesions involving the posterior part of the superior temporal gyrus (Wernicke's area).

Other Aphasias

A distinct form of aphasia called *conduction aphasia* is characterized by an inability to repeat what is said, with preserved fluency and comprehension. Classic teaching states that the lesion responsible lies in the arcuate fasciculus, the white matter connections between Broca's

and Wernicke's areas. However, there is little anatomic evidence to support this idea, and in fact lesions involving the temporal or parietal lobes (but sparing Wernicke's area) can lead to this syndrome. Conduction aphasia patients also make many paraphasic errors, ones we all normally correct "on the fly" as we monitor our own speech, a function they cannot perform.

Lesions in the frontal lobe slightly superior to Broca's area can cause a nonfluent aphasia very similar to Broca's aphasia except that repetition is preserved, since the path between and including Broca's and Wernicke's areas is unaffected. Such a *transcortical motor aphasia* can also be caused by lesions in the supplementary motor area and in the anterior portions of the basal ganglia.

Similarly, a *transcortical sensory aphasia* is caused by lesions in the inferior portion of the left temporal lobe and is characterized by fluent speech with impaired comprehension but preserved repetition. Infarcts in the territory of the left posterior cerebral artery (PCA) and small temporal lobe hemorrhages and contusions are the commonest causes.

◆ KEY POINTS ◆

1. Conduction aphasia, primarily characterized by an inability to repeat, is caused by lesions involving the temporal and parietal lobes but sparing Wernicke's area.

2. Transcortical motor and sensory aphasias resemble Broca's and Wernicke's aphasias, respectively, except that repetition is preserved.

Global aphasia, typically caused by large dominant hemisphere lesions affecting the frontal and temporal lobes including Broca's and Wernicke's areas, results in problems with language production, comprehension, and repetition.

Subcortical aphasias are acquired language deficits associated with lesions in deep dominant hemisphere structures, such as the basal ganglia and thalamus. These typically do not fall easily into the aphasia classification given above, although more anterior subcortical lesions have a tendency to produce aphasias that resemble Broca's aphasia and more posterior lesions lead to aphasias that resemble Wernicke's. Often subcortical aphasias are accompanied by hypophonia of the voice.

Disorders of Written Communication

Reading and writing are commonly affected in all of the aphasias. Typically, reading parallels comprehension of spoken language, while writing parallels production of spoken language, although the respective difficulties with written language are typically much worse than those with spoken language. Thus Broca's patients may be able to understand simple commands by reading them, though they cannot read them aloud or write.

A unique syndrome called *alexia without agraphia*, or *pure alexia*, is characterized by an inability to read despite a preserved ability to write. This leads to the surprising finding that a patient may not be able to read back the words she has just successfully written. The responsible lesion is situated in the dominant occipital lobe but also involves the splenium of the corpus callosum. In this way the fibers connecting visual cortex (on either side) to Wernicke's area in the dominant hemisphere are interrupted, thus preventing input of language through visual means. A contralateral homonymous hemianopia is typically an associated finding.

APRAXIA

Apraxia is defined as an inability to carry out a learned motor task despite preservation of the primary functions needed to carry out the task, such as comprehension, motor ability, sensation, and coordination.

A patient with an apraxia, for example, might not be able to demonstrate how to hammer a nail, despite sufficient language comprehension to understand the command and sufficient motor strength, sensation in the hands, and coordination to carry out the command. It is as if the patient cannot imagine or execute the motor program for the task.

Terminology regarding different types of apraxias, including names such as *ideational*, *ideomotor*, and *limb-kinetic*, is confusing. It is more enlightening simply to describe what the patient can and cannot do. In one type of apraxia, patients can recognize when others are carrying out the task correctly rather than incorrectly, but cannot perform the motor task themselves. Sometimes these patients can carry out the task with the actual objects given to them (e.g., using a real hammer and nail) but cannot mimic the task without the actual objects. In another type of apraxia, patients cannot even recognize when others are carrying out the task correctly.

Diagnosis

There are three basic ways to test for apraxia: asking patients to pretend they are performing an action, to mimic the examiner performing an action, or to use actual objects in performing an action. Examples of bedside tests include asking the patient to wave goodbye, salute, brush his teeth, or comb his hair. Two-handed tasks, such as hammering in a nail or slicing a loaf of bread, are more demanding. Some patients who have a specific form of apraxia involving oral movements may be unable to demonstrate whistling or blowing out a match. Many patients with apraxia will have a tendency to use their limb as object (e.g., running their fingers through their hair when asked to demonstrate how to use a comb).

Etiology

Apraxias are typically associated with either frontal or parietal lesions in the dominant hemisphere. Frontal lesions typically cause apraxias in which patients are able to recognize the task done correctly by others but cannot perform it themselves, whereas parietal lesions typically result in apraxias in which patients cannot recognize the task done correctly.

◆ KEY POINTS ◆

1. Apraxia is the inability to perform a learned motor task despite preservation of the necessary basic motor, sensory, and cognitive capacities.

2. Examples of bedside tests for apraxia include asking a patient to mimic the motions necessary to brush her teeth, comb her hair, hammer in a nail, or slice a loaf of bread.

3. Apraxia is typically caused by lesions in the frontal or parietal lobes of the dominant hemisphere.

AGNOSIA

Agnosia refers to an inability to recognize objects through one or more sensory modalities, despite the preserved functioning of those primary sensory modalities.

Diagnosis

A patient with visual agnosia, for example, might not be able to recognize objects placed in his vision, though all other aspects of his vision, such as acuity and fields, are intact. The same patient would be able to recognize those objects when allowed to touch them. With his vision, he might be able to describe specific features of the object, but he would not be able to recognize the object as a whole.

Etiology

Agnosias are typically caused by lesions in the sensory association areas of the brain, processing areas that lie next to the primary sensory areas and are responsible for integrating primary sensory information into higher-order complex forms. For example, the visual association area lies in the occipitotemporal region anterior and inferior to the primary visual cortex and is responsible for the recognition of objects using primary visual information. Lesions here cause a visual agnosia. A specific form called *prosopagnosia*, an inability to recognize faces, can occur with right hemisphere or bilateral lesions in the visual association area.

◆ KEY POINTS ◆

1. Agnosia is the inability to recognize objects despite preservation of the basic sensory modalities being used.
2. Agnosia is typically caused by lesions in the sensory association areas.

GERSTMANN'S SYNDROME

Lesions in the inferior parietal lobule of the dominant hemisphere, and specifically in the angular gyrus (see Fig. 11–1), cause *Gerstmann's syndrome*, a constellation of problems in higher cortical function. These are agraphia, the inability to write; acalculia, the inability to

calculate; right-left confusion; and finger agnosia, the inability to recognize one's own or the examiner's individual fingers. One explanation is that this area of the parietal lobe is responsible for the symbolic representation of body parts as well as orthographic and numerical symbols.

◆ KEY POINTS ◆

1. Gerstmann's syndrome is characterized by four elements: agraphia, acalculia, right-left confusion, and finger agnosia.
2. Gerstmann's syndrome is typically caused by lesions in the angular gyrus of the dominant hemisphere.

NEGLECT

There are times when it seems that all interesting higher cortical functions reside in the dominant hemisphere. Neglect, however, one of the most fascinating cortical disorders, is usually the result of damage to the nondominant (usually right) hemisphere.

Neglect is directed inattention, or a relative lack of attention, paid to one hemispace. Patients with neglect will tend to be less aware (or completely unaware) of objects or actions in one side of the world (usually the left). It is not that they have a hemianopia and cannot see that side, or a primary motor or sensory deficit for that side; rather, they have decreased attention toward the left side.

Diagnosis

Those with the most severe forms of neglect completely ignore the left side and deny that such a side even exists. They may leave their left side ungroomed, unshaven, and undressed; they may leave food on the left side of their plate untouched. They may deny that they have a left hand, and when confronted with it, may claim that it is actually the examiner's. When asked to describe their surroundings or draw a picture, they may omit items on the left side (Fig. 11–2).

Patients with milder neglect may not have such gross abnormalities but may perform actions with their left side only with encouragement or after repeated prod-

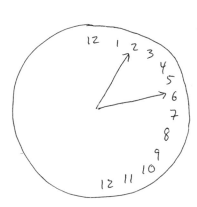

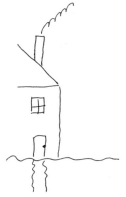

Figure 11–2 Examples of drawings demonstrating neglect of the left side.

ding. When asked to bisect a line, they may err off toward the right. When asked to cross out letters scattered across a page, they may leave some on the left side unmarked.

The most sensitive sign of neglect, which may be the only finding seen in patients with the mildest form, is extinction to double simultaneous stimulation. This phenomenon occurs when sensory stimuli applied singly to either side are properly felt, but when both sides are stimulated simultaneously only the non-neglected side is felt. Extinction may exist with tactile, visual, or auditory stimulation.

Etiology

Neglect is typically caused by lesions in the right hemisphere, particularly the right frontal or parietal lobes. It is most commonly seen as an acute finding after a stroke, though other pathologies in these areas can cause a similar clinical syndrome. Lesions in the right frontal lobe may cause more of a motor neglect, in which the patient has a tendency to not use the left side for motor actions, whereas lesions in the right parietal lobe may cause more of a sensory neglect, in which stimuli from the left side tend to be ignored.

◆ KEY POINTS ◆

1. Neglect is directed inattention, or a relative lack of attention, paid to one hemispace, usually the left.

2. Patients with severe neglect may fail to describe objects on the left, may fail to dress or shave their left side, or may even deny that their left arm is theirs.

3. Those with milder forms may not bisect lines or cancel out letters properly, or may exhibit extinction to double simultaneous stimulation.

4. Neglect is usually caused by lesions in the right frontal or parietal lobe.

OTHER NONDOMINANT HEMISPHERE SYNDROMES

The semantic elements of language (those associated purely with meaning) reside in the dominant (usually left) hemisphere, as described in the discussion on aphasias above. However, some of the other elements of successful oral communication, such as changing the inflection of one's voice when asking a question or when making an angry statement, reside in the nondominant (usually right) hemisphere. These elements are collectively referred to as *prosody*, and patients with right hemisphere lesions may have difficulty with this part of communication. Some may have difficulty applying the proper inflection to their own speech output, for example, and sound fairly monotone. Others may have difficulty understanding the speech inflections of those speaking to them, and cannot distinguish between a statement said to them in anger or in jest.

Some patients with right hemisphere lesions have a tendency to be unaware of their deficits, a condition termed *anosognosia*. A patient with a complete left hemiplegia, for example, may insist on immediate discharge from the hospital because he feels nothing is wrong. A patient with a dense left hemianopia may wonder why she keeps bumping into others since she notices nothing wrong with her vision. As expected, these patients tend to have more difficult and unsuccessful rehabilitations.

12 Dementia

Dementia is a common cause of morbidity and mortality in the elderly and has many different causes. It implies an intellectual and cognitive deterioration of sufficient severity to interfere with normal functioning. Memory, orientation, visuospatial perception, language, and higher executive functions (planning, organizing, and sequencing) may be impaired in dementia.

The term *delirium* or *acute confusional state* implies a global disturbance of mental functions, in general reversible, accompanied by altered level of consciousness.

EPIDEMIOLOGY

Dementia is most common in the elderly but can occur at a younger age (particularly in those with a hereditary component). Approximately 5% of people between ages 65 and 70 have dementia; this increases to more than 45% above age 85. Alzheimer's disease accounts for 50% to 70% of cases of dementia. Cerebrovascular disease accounts for about 15% to 20%, and the other causes presented in Table 12–1 account for most of the rest. Dementia has a considerable social cost (over $50 billion in the United States every year).

CLINICAL MANIFESTATION

There is a known cognitive decline with old age, and sometimes the differentiation between a dementing illness and age-related cognitive decline is difficult. In general, most patients with dementia start having problems with short-term memory, followed by an indolent deterioration of cognitive functions that may involve language, praxis, and so forth. Many dementing illnesses manifest characteristic symptoms and clinical findings that are helpful in establishing an etiologic diagnosis.

DIAGNOSIS

The initial recognition of dementia is difficult. Normal aging and depression can mimic some of its features. Rarely, the patient is aware of cognitive deterioration; in most cases, the family brings the patient to the doctor months or years after problems have started. The most important information in the diagnosis of dementia is the clinical history (including reports by relatives) and the physical exam (with a very detailed mental status examination). Then, the diagnosis of the cause of dementia consists of matching the major clinical features of the individual patient with characteristics of known dementing illnesses.

The use of laboratory tests depends on the clinical history and exam, the tentative diagnosis, and the possibility of finding reversible causes. Table 12–2 summarizes some tests to consider. Most are used to rule out reversible causes of dementia.

TABLE 12–1

Causes of Dementia

Degenerative
  Alzheimer's disease
  Huntington's disease
  Parkinson's disease
  Lewy body dementia
  Pick's disease
  Progressive supranuclear palsy
  Amyotrophic lateral sclerosis with dementia
  Olivopontocerebellar atrophy
  Frontotemporal dementia associated with
    chromosome 17 (FTD-17)

Metabolic
  Wilson's disease
  Hypothyroidism
  Vitamin B_{12} deficiency
  Hypercalcemia
  Addison's disease

Lipid storage diseases and leukodystrophies

Toxic
  Drug intoxication
  Alcohol
  Arsenic, mercury, and lead intoxication

Infectious
  Creutzfeldt-Jakob disease
  HIV
  Syphilis
  Subacute sclerosis panencephalitis (post-measles)

Neoplastic and paraneoplastic

Vascular
  Vascular dementia
  Vasculitis

Hydrocephalus

Traumatic
  Severe head injury
  Boxer's encephalopathy (punch drunk)
  Chronic subdural hematoma

Undetermined

Mixed (Alzheimer's plus vascular)

TABLE 12–2

Tests to Consider in a Patient with Dementia

Hematologic screening, including erythrocyte
  sedimentation rate

Vitamin B_{12} and folate

Blood calcium

Liver function tests, including ammonia

Electrolytes

Serum urea nitrogen and creatinine levels

Infectious workup, including syphilis, HIV, tuberculosis,
  etc.

EEG: Should not be routinely ordered in a dementia
  assessment. Its use is justified when the patient has
  evidence of fluctuations in cognitive status that
  could represent seizures. The EEG may be useful at
  the initial presentation in patients with suspected
  Creutzfeldt-Jakob disease (CJD).

CT or MRI of the brain (rule out structural
  abnormalities such as tumor, subdural hematoma,
  and hydrocephalus, and evaluate cortical atrophy)

Neuropsychologic assessment: Useful in early stages to
  establish the diagnosis of dementia and to use as a
  comparison tool in the progression of the disease

Brain biopsy: Only indicated in specific cases such as
  CJD, HIV, CNS vasculitis, and so on, to confirm the
  diagnosis and find or exclude possible treatable
  causes

◆ KEY POINTS ◆

1. Symptoms and signs of dementia include memory loss, abnormalities of speech, difficulties with problem-solving and abstract thinking, impaired judgment, personality changes, and emotional lability.

2. The diagnosis of the cause of dementia requires a detailed history and neurologic and physical examination.

CAUSES OF DEMENTIA

Alzheimer's Disease

In 1907, Alois Alzheimer, a German clinician and neuropathologist, published the landmark case of a 51-year-old woman with deterioration of her mental state. Her autopsy disclosed the classic pathology of Alzheimer's disease (AD): neurofibrillary tangles and senile plaques in the cerebral neocortex and hippocampus.

Epidemiology

Nearly 4% of people older than 65 years have severe Alzheimer's disease and are incapacitated. Recent estimates suggest that more than 2 million people have AD in the United States alone. Because of increased life expectancy, the population at risk for AD is the fastest growing segment of society. Annually, approximately 100,000 people die from Alzheimer's disease and more than $25 billion is spent on the institutional care of patients with AD.

Etiology and Risk Factors

Many factors are associated with an increased frequency of AD, including age, female sex, history of severe head trauma, and Down syndrome.

There are also many putative genetic risk factors. The gene for ApoE4 (chromosome 19) has been shown to be associated with both early- and late-onset AD of both sporadic and familial varieties. Early-onset AD has been associated with mutations in the amyloid precursor protein (APP) on chromosome 21, and presenilin 1 (PS1) and presenilin 2 (PS2) on chromosomes 14 and 1, respectively. There are more than 65 mutations described in these genes. Another mutation in a gene on chromosome 12 that encodes α_2-macroglobulin has been associated with AD. The ApoE alleles and the α_2-macroglobulin mutation predispose individuals to early onset of sporadic AD and even more to late-onset AD. The other mutations in APP, PS1, and PS2 are associated with early onset of the disease, in the third through sixth decades.

Amyloid-beta protein precursor (AbPP) mutations may cause an increased amyloid-beta (Ab) production with subsequent aggregation in the cells. This mutation changes the normal structure of the protein, altering its recognition by metabolizing enzymes like alpha-secretase and utilizing alternative pathways for degradation, leading to a progressive accumulation of the peptide. Other pathophysiologic mechanisms have been described, including inflammatory, oxidative, metabolic, nutritional, and immune.

Clinical Manifestations

"Doctor, my mother is 75 years old and over the last 3 years I have noted that she is having more difficulty with her memory. She remembers her marriage 50 years ago but she does not remember that we were here yesterday. She constantly asks the same questions and forgets my answers. She is unable to balance her check book and yesterday she could not find the way home from the drugstore." This history illustrates characteristic features of AD. At the beginning of the illness, the exam shows no difficulty with language, reasoning, or in performance of normal social and personal behaviors. Only those close to the patient notice small slip-ups that suggest that something is wrong (becoming lost while driving, misplacement of objects, the kitchen left unattended, missed appointments, loss of social and interpersonal interactions). Later, the patient has more difficulty with activities of daily life.

As the disease progresses, other aspects of cognitive function are lost, including the ability to speak, understand, think, and make decisions. Characteristically, in contrast to patients with vascular dementia, elementary neurologic functions (motor, visual, somatosensory, and gait) remain normal until very late in the disease. Psychiatric manifestations are common at this time: personality changes (apathetic or impulsive), aggressive behavior (physical or verbal), paranoid thoughts and delusions (persecution, things being stolen), sleep disturbances ("sundowning" is used to describe worsening psychiatric manifestations during the night), hallucinations (uncommon and in general a side effect of medications), and depression. The course is relentlessly progressive, and the patient usually succumbs over 5 to 10 years due to a combination of neurologic and medical problems.

Diagnosis

Except for brain biopsy, there are no tests that definitively establish the diagnosis of AD in living patients. The diagnosis is suggested by the clinical features and by the insidiously progressive course. Investigations are designed to exclude other causes of dementia (see Table 12–2). Elevated Tau protein and low Ab-42 levels in the cerebrospinal fluid (CSF) have been suggested as early diagnostic markers for AD. Magnetic resonance imaging (MRI)-based volumetric measurements may show reduction of up to 40% in the size of the hippocampus, amygdala, and thalamus. Functional neuroimaging such as PET (positron emission tomography) and SPECT (single-photon emission computed tomography), used to quantify cerebral metabolism and blood flow, may help to differentiate AD from other dementias. In Alzheimer's disease, PET and SPECT scans show a nonspecific bilateral temporoparietal hypometabolism.

Pathology

The major pathologic features of AD are brain atrophy, senile plaques, and neurofibrillary tangles (NFTs), associated with substantial loss of neurons in the cerebral cortex and gliosis. NFTs represent intracellular accumulation of phosphorylated Tau protein. Senile plaques are extracellular deposits of amyloid surrounded by dystrophic axons.

Management

At present there is no satisfactory treatment for patients with Alzheimer's disease.

Therapy consists of the following:

- *Preventing associated symptoms:* Treatment of depression, agitation, sleep disorders, hallucinations, and delusions.
- *Preventing progression:* This includes therapy with acetylcholinesterase inhibitors such as donepezil or rivastigmine.
- *Prophylaxis:* No data from randomized clinical trials are available. Use of vitamin E, nonsteroidal anti-inflammatory drugs (NSAIDs), and estrogens has been proposed.

Table 12–3 provides information regarding therapy of AD and other dementias.

◆ KEY POINTS ◆

1. Alzheimer's disease is the most common neurodegenerative disease of the brain and accounts for 50% to 70% of all instances of dementia.
2. Risk factors for developing AD include older age, female sex, head trauma, and family history.

3. Potentially treatable causes of dementia should be excluded through laboratory testing and brain imaging.
4. The average length of time from onset of symptoms until diagnosis is 2 to 3 years. The average duration from diagnosis to nursing-home placement is 3 to 6 years. AD patients spend 3 years in nursing homes before death. Thus, the total duration of AD is roughly 9 to 12 years.

Vascular Dementia

This dementia (previously referred to as multi-infarct dementia) may develop in patients with cerebrovascular disease. There are two recognized types: macrovascular, related to large infarcts; and microvascular, in which the pathophysiologic mechanism of brain injury is subcortical ischemia associated with cerebral small vessel disease (lacunes or deep white matter changes on MRI). Vascular dementia has the risk factors of cerebrovascular disease, including hypertension, diabetes, age, embolic sources, and extensive large artery atherosclerosis. It is not infrequent for vascular dementia and Alzheimer's disease to coexist in the same patient.

Clinical Manifestations and Diagnosis

The criteria for diagnosis of vascular dementia include presence of dementia and two or more of the following: focal neurologic signs on physical examination; onset that was abrupt, stepwise, or stroke related; or brain imaging study showing multiple strokes, lacunes, or extensive deep white matter changes. Most patients with vascular dementia are hypertensive or diabetic. The diagnosis requires investigation of the cause of stroke. Cardiac and hypercoagulable workup should be considered in selected cases.

Management

The prevention and treatment of vascular dementia are essentially the same as prevention and treatment of stroke (see Table 12–3 and Chapter 14).

TABLE 12–3

Dementia Therapy

	Dose	Comments
Alzheimer's disease		
Donepezil (Aricept)	5–10 mg po qlts	Equal efficacy and fewer side effects than tacrine. Rare: hepatic toxicity. Common: diarrhea and abdominal cramps
Rivastigmine (Exelon)	6–12 mg/day, given po bid; start 1.5 mg po bid	GI disturbances during dose adjustment. Rare: hepatic toxicity. Recently approved by FDA.
Tacrine	10 mg po qid	Hepatic toxicity. Check ALT every 2 weeks during dosage titration.
Ibuprofen	400 mg po tid	Targeting the anti-inflammatory theory of AD. Not proven different from placebo in recent studies
Vitamin E	800–2000 IU po daily	Mild anticoagulant effect, particularly with patients on coumadin.
Conjugated estrogens	0.625 mg po daily	Women only. Not proven in recent clinical trials to alter the course of the disease.
Vascular dementia		
Antihypertensive medications	Any	Maintain systolic BP below 160 and diastolic between 85 and 95. Treatments that lower diastolic BP may worsen cognitive function
Warfarin	Variable	Check INR and maintain value between 2 and 3. Indicated in patient with atrial fibrillation and strokes.
Aspirin	81–325 po mg qD	Consider warfarin if atrial fibrillation is present.
Clopidogrel (Plavix)	75 mg po qD	Can produce TTP. Can be used in combination with aspirin.
Dipyridamole and aspirin (Aggrenox)	1 capsule po bid	Same indications as aspirin.
Vitamin E	800–2000 IU daily	Mild anticoagulant effect, particularly with patients on coumadin.

ALT, alanine aminotransferase; BP, blood pressure; INR, international normalized ratio; TTP, thrombotic thrombocytopenic purpura.

Dementias Associated with Extrapyramidal Features

This group of dementias includes dementia with Lewy bodies, progressive supranuclear palsy, corticobasal degeneration, striatonigral degeneration, Huntington's disease, and Wilson's disease.

Dementia with Lewy Bodies

The clinical picture is that of a parkinsonian dementia syndrome with visual hallucinations. Sometimes it is very difficult to differentiate this from a Parkinson's patient who develops dementia.

Clinical Manifestations

The major features are cognitive impairment (severe visuospatial perception and visual memory problems), marked fluctuations of alertness, prominent visual hallucinations (up to 80% of cases) and delusions, extrapyramidal symptoms, and extraordinary sensitivity to neuroleptics.

Diagnosis

The pathologic hallmark is the Lewy body (also found in Parkinson's disease), an eosinophilic intracellular inclusion of alpha synuclein found mainly in neurons of cortical, subcortical, and brainstem structures. There are also varying degrees of AD-type abnormalities such as NFTs and senile plaques.

Management

Treatment of the parkinsonian syndrome may worsen neuropsychiatric dysfunction, and treatment of the neuropsychiatric disorder may exacerbate the parkinsonian syndrome. Low doses of atypical neuroleptics such as risperidone and clozapine have been used to treat behavioral symptoms.

Progressive Supranuclear Palsy

Also known as the Steele-Richardson-Olszewski syndrome, progressive supranuclear palsy (PSP) may account for 2% to 3% of dementias. No clear predisposing or genetic factors have been identified.

Clinical Manifestations

The main features are supranuclear ocular palsy (mainly failure of vertical gaze), dysarthria, dysphagia, extrapyramidal rigidity, gait ataxia, and dementia. In the early stages of PSP, falls and gait abnormalities are prominent. Dementia may occur early or develop later. Frontal lobe abnormalities predominate. Patients become apathetic and talk and act less. In early stages, PSP may be mistaken for AD.

Diagnosis

The pathology shows atrophy of the dorsal midbrain, globus pallidus, and subthalamic nucleus. NFTs, neuronal loss, and gliosis in many subcortical structures are characteristic. The course is progressive, with a median survival of 6 to 10 years.

Huntington's Disease

Huntington's disease (HD) is an autosomal dominant neurodegenerative disorder with predominant basal ganglia abnormalities.

Clinical Manifestations

Symptoms usually appear between age 35 and 45 and include the triad of chorea, behavioral changes or personality disorder (frequently obsessive-compulsive disorder), and dementia. The three may occur together at onset or one may precede the others by years.

Diagnosis

Diagnosis is by family history, clinical signs, atrophy of the caudate on brain imaging, and the demonstration of more than 40 CAG repeats in chromosome 4.

Pathology

Pathologic examination shows severe destruction of the caudate and putamen (striatal and nigral GABA-ergic neurons), and loss of neurons in the cerebral cortex (layer 3). HD is linked to chromosome 4p16.3 on the HD gene, encoding for a protein named *huntingtin*. The mutation produces an unstable CAG repeat. This induces aberrant processing of cell proteins with formation of deposits in the nucleus and activation of intracellular mechanisms of cell death.

Management

Pharmacologic management of dementia and chorea often involves dopaminergic antagonists, including neuroleptic drugs, but is far from adequate. Genetic counseling is fundamental.

◆ **KEY POINTS** ◆

1. Huntington's disease is characterized by chorea, dementia, and personality and behavioral changes.
2. Death occurs 10 to 20 years after onset.
3. Suicide is not rare in at-risk and early-onset HD patients.

Parkinson's Disease

Parkinson's disease (PD) may produce subcortical dementia. Cognitive impairment develops in about 30% of patients with idiopathic PD. The distinction from other types of dementia is based on the natural history and the presence of associated symptoms. The clinical manifestations include those of subcortical dementia with marked psychomotor involvement.

Frontotemporal Dementia

Frontotemporal dementia (FTD) is a primary degenerative dementia characterized by significant alteration in personality and social behavior.

Clinical Manifestations

Patients neglect social and personal responsibilities, present failure in judgment, and show defective sequencing and organization. FTDs include Pick's disease, FTD and motor neuron disease, FTD and parkinsonism linked to chromosome 17 (FTD-17), progressive nonfluent aphasia, semantic dementia, and progressive apraxia.

Pick's disease is a rare form of progressive dementia characterized by personality change, speech disturbance, inattentiveness, and sometimes extrapyramidal signs. The diagnosis is made by clinical history and the presence of circumscribed frontotemporal lobar atrophy. Argyrophilic round intraneuronal inclusions (Pick bodies) are the characteristic pathologic changes. Abnormal Tau protein with Tau-positive inclusions are found in neurons and glial cells. Senile plaques are not present.

◆ **KEY POINTS** ◆

1. FTDs are rare.
2. Lobar atrophy is characteristic.
3. Personality changes early in the disease are characteristic.

Dementias Caused by Infectious Agents

Prion-Related Diseases

Prion-related diseases include Creutzfeldt-Jakob disease, or CJD (familial and sporadic); Gerstmann-Sträussler-Scheinker syndrome; and fatal familial insomnia.

The so-called spongiform encephalopathies are a group of disorders characterized by spongy degeneration, neuronal loss, gliosis, and astrocytic proliferation resulting from the accumulation in the brain of a mutated protease-resistant prion protein.

CJD is the most common of these disorders. It is characterized by a rapidly progressive dementia with pyramidal signs, myoclonus, cerebellar or extrapyramidal signs, and periodic sharp waves in the electroencephalogram (EEG). MRI with DWI (diffusion-weighted images) may show evolving cortical and basal ganglia abnormalities during the course of the disease. CSF is typically normal, but the presence of protein 14-3-3 is highly sensitive and specific for CJD. There is no therapy. This syndrome evolves over weeks to months, and death usually occurs within one year.

◆ KEY POINTS ◆

1. CJD is rare.
2. CJD presents as a rapidlic progressive dementia with focal neurologic signs and myoclonus.
3. EEG and MRI are not diagnostic, but in the setting of the appropriate clinical history they become more specific.

HIV-Associated Dementia Complex

Most patients with human immunodeficiency virus (HIV) disease have central nervous system (CNS) involvement. The virus not only can produce encephalitis, but also makes the individual susceptible to CNS infections such as toxoplasmosis, tuberculosis, and syphilis, which can cause dementia as well. HIV-associated dementia complex is a clinical entity recognized in HIV patients (usually with low CD4 counts) and is characterized by progressive deterioration of cognitive function.

Clinical Manifestations

Patients report memory problems, difficulty with concentration, and poor attention. The pathophysiologic bases for this cognitive impairment have not been clarified.

Diagnosis

MRI usually shows cortical and subcortical atrophy.

Management

Zidovudine (AZT) is controversial. Currently, selegiline and memantine (an NMDA antagonist) are being evaluated. High-dose antiretroviral therapy may be helpful in retarding cognitive loss.

◆ KEY POINTS ◆

1. HIV-associated dementia is common in HIV patients with low CD4 counts.
2. Therapy includes AZT, selegiline, and memantine.

Metabolic Causes of Dementia

Vitamin B_{12} deficiency may present as a progressive dementing illness. However, there are usually many other neurologic features including dysfunction in the spinal cord (subacute combined degeneration) and peripheral nervous system, such that the diagnosis becomes clearer. The most common neurologic symptoms are those of neuropathy (paresthesias in hands and feet, sensory ataxia, visual loss, orthostatic hypotension) and memory loss. Systemic symptoms include anemia and sore tongue. Appropriate replacement of vitamin B_{12} should suffice in the treatment. Other metabolic causes of dementia are mentioned in Table 12–1.

13 Sleep Disorders

PHYSIOLOGY

Normal sleep is divided into two states: rapid eye movement (REM) and non-REM. REM sleep alternates with non-REM sleep in 90-minute cycles (Fig. 13–1), with vivid dreaming occurring during REM sleep. These sleep cycles are under cerebral influence. Thus, sleep medicine is an interdisciplinary specialty usually consisting of internists, pulmonary specialists, and neurologists. Polysomnography is the main tool that sleep specialists use in order to distinguish sleep states. Recordings are derived from electroencephalograms (EEG), electromyograms (EMG) to demonstrate muscle tone, and electro-oculograms to determine eye movements. In addition, other physiologic measures such as nasal and oral airflow, respiratory effort, and cardiac rhythm are monitored.

Using polysomnography, non-REM sleep is divided into four stages (I, II, III, and IV). During the awake state, the EEG usually shows an 8- to 13-Hz rhythm (alpha rhythm), predominantly in the posterior portions of the brain. Stage I sleep is characterized by diminished alpha rhythms that are replaced by 4- to 7-Hz activity with some 12- to 14-Hz activity. Stage II sleep is characterized by sleep spindles (bursts of 12- to 14-Hz activity) and K complexes (high-voltage waves of both positive and negative polarity, best seen in EEG leads at the vertex of the head). Stage III and stage IV sleep are characterized by the presence of slow-wave activity of 4 Hz or less (delta waves). Stage III is defined as 20% to 50% of a set period consisting of delta waves, and stage IV sleep occurs when greater than 50% of the set period is occupied by delta waves.

Normal people progress in an orderly fashion through the four stages of non-REM sleep, with stage IV (delta sleep) occurring 30 to 45 minutes after sleep onset. REM sleep occurs 60 to 90 minutes after sleep onset, and the EMG shows loss of tone in all muscles except for respiratory and ocular muscles. The EEG shows mixed frequencies, and respirations and heart rate are irregular. At the end of the REM sleep, the first cycle of sleep is completed. Thereafter, non-REM sleep continues to alternate with REM sleep for a total of four to six cycles through the night in a normal healthy young adult (see Fig. 13–1).

◆ KEY POINTS ◆

1. Sleep is divided into REM and non-REM sleep.

2. Non-REM sleep is divided into four stages (I, II, III, and IV).

3. REM sleep is characterized by loss of muscle tone except in the respiratory and eye muscles.

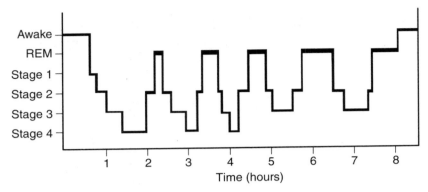

Figure 13–1   Stages of sleep. REM sleep and the four stages of non-REM sleep alternate throughout the night in cycles that last approximately 90 minutes. There are typically four to six cycles each night in a healthy young adult.

SLEEP DISORDERS

The International Classification of Sleep Disorders defines four major categories of sleep disorders: dyssomnias, parasomnias, sleep disorders associated with medical and psychiatric conditions, and proposed sleep disorders. The more common sleep disorders from the first three categories are covered below.

Dyssomnias

Dyssomnias are primary sleep disorders that produce either difficulty initiating and maintaining sleep (insomnia) or excessive daytime sleepiness. A detailed history including medications, caffeine use, alcohol consumption, and drug use can often reveal the cause of insomnia.

Narcolepsy is a disorder of unknown etiology characterized by excessive daytime sleepiness often associated with cataplexy and other REM sleep phenomena such as hypnagogic hallucinations or sleep paralysis. The onset of narcolepsy is typically between 15 and 25 years of age, with a family history in two-thirds of cases. The cardinal feature of narcolepsy is excessive daytime sleepiness that can occur at inappropriate times or places. The naps usually last from a few minutes to 15 to 30 minutes and are remarkably refreshing. Patients can go on to develop cataplexy, which is a brief loss in muscle tone in which the patient will fall to the ground or the head may slump forward for a few

seconds. These attacks are often triggered by emotion such as laughter or anger. Consciousness is preserved, but prolonged episodes may be followed immediately by REM sleep.

Hypnagogic hallucinations are hallucinations that occur at the beginning of sleep and can involve the visual, auditory, or vestibular system. These hallucinations are a manifestation of sudden onset of inappropriate REM sleep. Another feature of narcolepsy, sleep paralysis, is an inability to move voluntary muscles during sleep/wake transitions. This can occur normally on awakening from REM sleep, but patients with narcolepsy usually experience the sensation at sleep onset.

Diagnosis of narcolepsy can be made clinically with a history of excessive daytime sleepiness associated with cataplexy. In those with an unclear history, polysomnography will typically show a short latency to sleep onset and sleep-onset REM. Treatment is with stimulants such as pemoline or methylphenidate. Clomipramine, a tricyclic antidepressant, is used to treat cataplexy.

Another disorder in the family of dyssomnias is obstructive sleep apnea, which is characterized by repetitive episodes of upper airway obstruction that occur during sleep. Other cardinal features include oxygen desaturation during the apneic spell, sleep disruption, and excessive daytime sleepiness. In severe cases, patients can fall asleep at inappropriate times such as driving or while at work. Diagnosis requires polysomnography throughout the night in order to measure degree of sleep disruption, oxygen desaturation, and number of apneas. Treatment is with nasal continuous positive airway pressure (CPAP), which helps maintain upper airway patency during sleep. Also, alcohol and sedating drugs that can decrease upper airway tone should be discontinued. Weight loss may be beneficial in reducing symptoms, since obesity is a strong risk factor for obstructive sleep apnea. Additionally, surgical treatment may be indicated if there is excessive tissue, such as enlarged tonsils, in the posterior pharynx.

Restless legs syndrome is another dyssomnia characterized by disagreeable leg sensations, usually prior to sleep onset, that cause an almost irresistible urge to move the legs. All patients with restless legs syndrome also suffer from periodic limb movement disorder, but some patients can suffer from the latter without having the former illness. Patients with periodic limb movement disorder have recurrent periodic leg jerks involving the flexor muscles of the legs. These twitches can occur every 20 to 40 seconds throughout the night and are usually noticed by the bed partner. Both of these limb disorders can be caused by metabolic abnormalities such as chronic alcohol use, uremia, or iron deficiency. Treatment is with dopamine agonists or benzodiazepines such as clonazepam.

◆ KEY POINTS ◆

1. Dyssomnias are primary sleep disorders that produce either difficulty initiating and maintaining sleep (insomnia) or excessive daytime sleepiness.
2. Narcolepsy is characterized by excessive daytime sleepiness often associated with cataplexy.
3. Narcolepsy is treated with pemoline or methylphenidate.
4. Obstructive sleep apnea is characterized by repetitive episodes of upper airway obstruction.
5. Obstructive sleep apnea is treated with nasal CPAP or surgery.

---

6. Restless legs syndrome is characterized by disagreeable leg sensations causing an almost irresistible urge to move the legs.

Parasomnias

Parasomnias are undesirable events that occur during sleep or are exacerbated by sleep. The more common parasomnias are sleepwalking, sleep terrors, nightmares, sleep bruxism, and sleep paralysis. Sleepwalking consists of complex behaviors initiated during slow-wave sleep and results in walking during sleep. Patients are in a confused state and can perform complex, automatic acts. Sleep terrors are characterized by sudden arousal from slow-wave sleep with a scream or cry accompanied by automatic and behavioral manifestations of intense fear. Nightmares are frightening dreams that occur during REM sleep and usually awaken the sleeper. Sleep bruxism is a stereotyped movement disorder characterized by grinding or clenching teeth during sleep. This is a common disorder that can result in disrupted sleep, damaged teeth, morning headaches, and temporomandibular joint dysfunction. A nocturnal tooth guard can alleviate symptoms. Sleep paralysis consists of a period of inability to perform voluntary movements at either sleep onset (hypnagogic) or upon awakening during the night or in the morning (hypnopompic).

Sleep Disorders Associated with Medical or Psychiatric Conditions

Sleep disorders occur during many psychiatric illnesses. For example, in patients with depression, there is often difficulty initiating and maintaining sleep, with early morning awakening. Patients with mania may have prolonged periods of inability to sleep. Medical conditions

---

◆ KEY POINTS ◆

1. Parasomnias are undesirable events that occur during sleep or are exacerbated by sleep.
2. Common parasomnias are sleepwalking, sleep terrors, nightmares, sleep bruxism, and sleep paralysis.

such as epilepsy are often exacerbated by sleep disturbances, and neurologic degenerative processes such as Parkinson's disease may have associated disrupted sleep patterns secondary to rigidity and tremor. Other medical conditions, such as pain from arthritis or peptic ulcer disease, and paroxysmal nocturnal dyspnea from congestive heart failure, can result in nocturnal arousal and disrupted sleep patterns. Therefore, a complete medical history is important in all patients who present with complaints of sleep disruption.

14 Vascular Disease

Stroke is the third leading cause of death in the United States, surpassed only by heart disease and cancer. Each year, approximately 750,000 people in the United States will have a stroke, and one-third to one-fourth of these patients will die from complications of their stroke. Furthermore, stroke is associated with significant morbidity characterized by disability, loss of independence, and emotional impact.

Risk factors for stroke include older age, male sex, family history, hypertension, diabetes, smoking, hypercholesterolemia, heavy alcohol use, and cardiac or peripheral vascular disease. Race is correlated with an increased risk of particular types of stroke. For example, Caucasian men have an increased risk of extracranial occlusive disease causing stroke compared with African Americans and Asians, who have a higher risk of intracranial stenosis and intracerebral hemorrhage.

Stroke is caused by acute damage to the nervous system caused by an abnormality of the blood supply that results in either ischemia or hemorrhage. Ischemia is the cause of approximately 80% of strokes, with hemorrhage responsible for the remaining 20%. If symptoms are brief (less than 30 minutes), the term *transient ischemic attack* (TIA) is often used. Symptoms that persist for greater than 24 hours are referred to as a *stroke*, and symptoms lasting from 30 minutes to 24 hours are referred to by some physicians as a *reversible ischemic neurologic deficit* (RIND). However, this labeling scheme is arbitrary and somewhat meaningless, because there is no clear clinical correlate of the specific time intervals.

Furthermore, because TIA is associated with a high risk of developing a future stroke, all patients with TIA, RIND, or strokes must be investigated for an underlying correctable etiology of their symptoms.

BRAIN ISCHEMIA

Ischemic stroke is caused by a lack of blood flow to the brain. It can be subdivided further into three different mechanisms: thrombosis, embolism, and decreased perfusion.

Thrombosis

Thrombosis refers to an obstruction of blood flow due to a localized occlusion within a blood vessel. The most common cause of thrombus formation is atherosclerotic disease that mainly affects the larger extracranial and intracranial blood vessels. Other sources of thrombus include primary hematologic diseases such as a systemic hypercoagulable state or thrombocytosis. In children, especially African American children, sickle cell disease is an important cause of thrombotic stroke. Other causes of thrombosis include fibromuscular dysplasia (caused by hyperplasia of the media layer of the blood vessel wall), arteritis, and arterial dissection. Clinically, neurologic symptoms tend to evolve over minutes or hours and can often have a stuttering or fluctuating course.

Embolism

An *embolus* is material that is formed elsewhere within the vascular system and travels to distant sites where the embolus becomes lodged, resulting in ischemia. Common sources of emboli are the heart (the most common); major arteries such as the aorta, carotid, or vertebral arteries; and systemic veins.

Emboli from the heart can originate from the heart valves or from tumors within the atrial or ventricular chambers. Emboli from arteries are composed of clot, clumps of platelets, or fragments of atherosclerotic plaques that break off and travel to more distal blood vessels. Systemic veins like those in the legs can be the source of clots. These clots can be the source of brain emboli if there is a defect in the heart such as a patent foramen ovale or atrial septal defect that allows the emboli to bypass the lungs and enter the left side of the heart and the peripheral circulation. This process is called *paradoxical embolism*. Clinically, embolic strokes tend to produce neurologic deficits that are maximal at onset.

Decreased Perfusion

Decreased systemic perfusion results from either systemic hypotension (hypovolemia or blood loss) or cardiac failure (caused by myocardial infarction or arrhythmia). The decreased perfusion usually results in a more generalized neurologic dysfunction in both cerebral hemispheres than that caused by an embolus or thrombus. Typically, the areas of the brain that are most vulnerable to hypoperfusion are the watershed or border-zone regions, which are areas of brain at the periphery of two different vascular territories.

◆ KEY POINTS ◆

1. Stroke can be either ischemic or hemorrhagic.

2. Ischemic stroke can be caused by embolism, thrombosis, or hypoperfusion.

3. A cardiac source is the most common cause of embolism.

4. Hypoperfusion results from hypovolemia or cardiac failure.

CEREBRAL HEMORRHAGE

Cerebral hemorrhages can be subdivided into two types: subarachnoid and intracerebral hemorrhage. Other hemorrhages such as epidural and subdural hematomas are discussed elsewhere (see Chapter 17). Hemorrhage leads to brain dysfunction through a variety of mechanisms, including destruction of tissue, mass effect, and compression of blood vessels leading to ischemia.

Subarachnoid Hemorrhage

Subarachnoid hemorrhage is most commonly caused by trauma (see Chapter 17) but can also be caused by bleeding from aneurysms or arteriovenous malformations. In the case of aneurysmal rupture, blood is rapidly released into the subarachnoid space, resulting in increased intracranial pressure. Aneurysms are commonly found at the junction between the anterior communicating artery and the anterior cerebral artery, at the bifurcation of the middle cerebral artery, in the posterior communicating artery, at the apex of the basilar artery, and at the origin of the posterior inferior cerebellar artery (Fig.

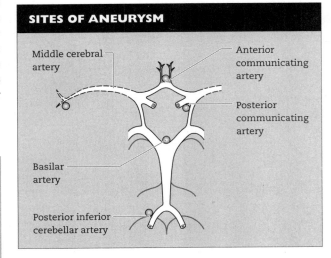

SITES OF ANEURYSM

Middle cerebral artery — Anterior communicating artery — Posterior communicating artery — Basilar artery — Posterior inferior cerebellar artery

Figure 14–1   Common sites of aneurysm in the circle of Willis. (Reproduced with permission from Ginsberg L. Lecture notes on neurology. Malden, MA: Blackwell Science, 1999:95.)

14–1). A sudden severe headache (commonly described as the worst headache of one's life) is the typical clinical presentation rather than focal neurologic deficits. As intracranial pressure rises, the patient may become lethargic or have other signs of altered mental state and may vomit.

Intracerebral Hemorrhage

Intracerebral or parenchymal hemorrhage is bleeding directly into the brain parenchyma itself. Trauma is the most common cause (see Chapter 17), followed by hypertension. Acute rises in blood pressure can lead to rupture of penetrating arteries. Also, long-standing hypertension damages small intracerebral arterioles and can result in leakage of blood. Other causes of intracerebral hemorrhage include anticoagulants such as heparin or warfarin, drug use such as cocaine or amphetamines, vascular malformations, and diseases affecting the blood vessel walls such as amyloid angiopathy. Other causes include hemorrhage into an underlying brain tumor.

The location of the hemorrhage and clinical history (i.e., history of anticoagulation or drug use) can be helpful in diagnosing the etiology of the hemorrhage. For example, hemorrhages caused by hypertension are most often found in the basal ganglia, thalamus, pons, and cerebellum (in order of decreasing frequency).

Lobar hemorrhages occur in the subcortical white matter in any cerebral lobe (frontal, temporal, parietal, and occipital). They can be caused by bleeding diathesis, trauma, an underlying lesion, and amyloid angiopathy that results from amyloid deposition in small arteries and arterioles in the leptomeninges and cerebral cortex, especially in the parietal and occipital lobes.

The clinical presentation of patients with intracerebral hemorrhage includes focal symptoms that may progress, headache, and loss of consciousness (with large hematomas). Herniation may also result from large intracerebral hemorrhages (see Chapter 17). Seizures are not common, but occur more frequently in patients with intracerebral hemorrhage than in other types of strokes. Additionally, hemorrhages may originate in the ventricles of the brain, in which case patients may present with headache, vomiting, decreased level of arousal, and neck stiffness.

◆ KEY POINTS ◆

1. Hemorrhagic strokes can be divided into subarachnoid and intracerebral hemorrhages.

2. Intracerebral hemorrhages are most commonly caused by trauma or chronic hypertension.

3. Hemorrhages related to hypertension are most commonly found in the basal ganglia, thalamus, pons, and cerebellum.

VASCULAR ANATOMY

To understand the varied clinical presentations of stroke, one must have a detailed knowledge of the anatomy and blood supply of the brain. Armed with this knowledge, one is able to accurately localize the lesion based on clinical features and examination findings. General neuroanatomic features and the vascular supply of the brain will be reviewed in order to understand the more commonly encountered stroke syndromes.

The arterial circulation to the brain is divided into the anterior and posterior circulation. *Anterior circulation* refers to the territory ultimately supplied by the carotid arteries, and *posterior circulation* refers to the territory ultimately supplied by the vertebral and basilar arteries (Fig. 14–2).

Anterior Circulation

The anterior circulation begins at the bifurcation of the common carotid artery to form the origin of the internal carotid artery. As the internal carotid artery enters the skull, it follows an S-shaped curve called the *siphon* that gives rise to its first branch, the ophthalmic artery. An embolus from the bifurcation of the carotid artery or from the siphon can travel to the ophthalmic artery, resulting in transient monocular blindness, also called *amaurosis fugax*. The internal carotid artery then penetrates the dura and gives rise to the anterior choroidal and posterior communicating arteries before it bifurcates to form the anterior cerebral artery, which courses anteriorly, and the middle cerebral artery, which courses laterally.

The anterior cerebral arteries supply the parasagittal cerebral cortex (Fig. 14–3) and are connected to each

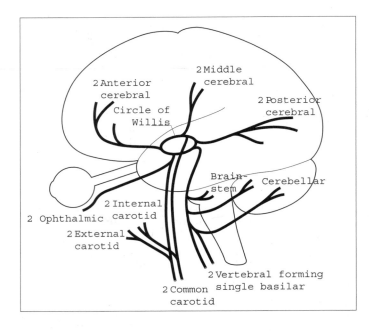

Figure 14–2 Schematic diagram of the vessels of the brain, including the anterior and posterior circulation. (Reproduced with permission from Wilkinson IMS. Essential neurology. Malden, MA: Blackwell Science, 1999:29.)

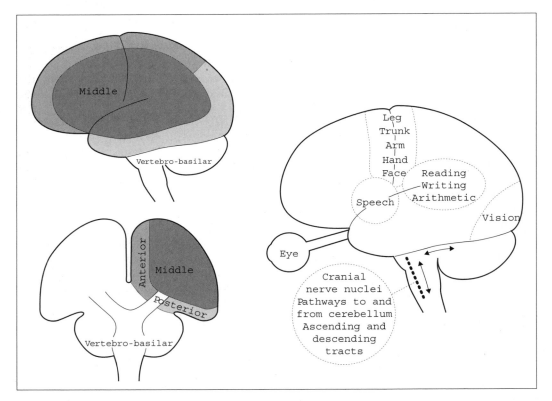

Figure 14–3 Arterial territories supplied by the anterior cerebral, middle cerebral, and posterior cerebral arteries, with corresponding localization of function. (Reproduced with permission from Wilkinson IMS. Essential neurology. Malden, MA: Blackwell Science, 1999:29.)

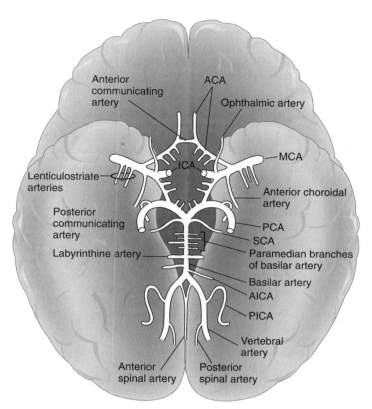

Figure 14–4 Arteries of the circle of Willis. ACA, anterior cerebral artery; AICA, anterior inferior cerebellar artery; ICA, internal cerebral artery; MCA, middle cerebral artery; PCA, posterior cerebral artery; PICA, posterior inferior cerebellar artery; SCA, superior cerebellar artery.

other via the anterior communicating artery (Fig. 14–4). The middle cerebral artery travels laterally and gives off the lenticulostriate artery branches that supply blood to the basal ganglia and internal capsule. As the middle cerebral artery continues through the sylvian fissure, it gives off several branches that supply the majority of the cerebral hemisphere (see Fig. 14–3).

Posterior Circulation

The posterior circulation is formed by a vertebral artery from each side. The two vertebral arteries unite in the midline at the junction of the medulla and pons to form the basilar artery. The vertebral arteries are the first branch from each subclavian artery and travel through the transverse foramina of the cervical vertebrae. The vertebral arteries give off posterior and anterior spinal artery branches and the posterior inferior cerebellar artery (PICA), which, as the name suggests, supplies blood to the posterior inferior cerebellum. The vertebral arteries then join, forming the basilar artery that gives off bilateral anterior inferior cerebellar arteries

(AICA) and superior cerebellar arteries (SCA). The basilar artery also gives off small branches that penetrate and supply the brainstem with blood. The basilar artery then divides at the junction of the pons and midbrain to form the posterior cerebral arteries (PCA) that give off branches to the midbrain and thalamus before supplying the occipital lobes and inferior portions of the temporal lobes (see Fig. 14–3).

The circle of Willis allows for communication of the blood supply between the anterior and posterior circulation via the posterior communicating arteries and allows for communication between the two sides of the anterior circulation via the anterior communicating artery (see Fig. 14–4).

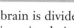

◆ KEY POINTS ◆

1. The arterial circulation to the brain is divided into the anterior and posterior circulation. The anterior circulation is the territory ulti-

> mately supplied by the carotid arteries, and the posterior circulation is the territory ultimately supplied by the vertebral and basilar arteries.
>
> 2. Amaurosis fugax usually results from an embolus to the ophthalmic artery.

COMMON STROKE SYNDROMES

Armed with this knowledge of neuroanatomy and the function of the nervous system (as discussed elsewhere, particularly Chapters 4 to 8 and 11), one can usually correlate the neurologic exam findings with one of seven common localization patterns.[1]

Left Hemisphere Lesion

This lesion can be caused by occlusion of the left internal carotid or middle cerebral artery. Clinical symptoms can include right-sided weakness and sensory loss, right visual field defect, inability to gaze to the right, and aphasia. The patient may also have impairment of reading, writing, and calculation. If the lesion is isolated to the anterior cerebral artery, the main finding will be right leg weakness.

Right Hemisphere Lesion

Similarly, the right hemisphere lesion results from occlusion of the right internal carotid or middle cerebral artery. Clinical symptoms can include left-sided weakness and sensory loss, inability to gaze to the left, neglect of the left visual space, cortical sensory defects (such as extinction of visual or tactile stimuli on the left side when presented simultaneously to both sides), difficulty drawing or copying, and aprosodic speech.

Left Posterior Cerebral Artery Lesion

Occlusion of the left PCA usually results in a right-sided visual field defect, sensory loss on the right side (if the thalamus is involved), difficulty naming colors presented visually, and alexia without agraphia (inability to read with preserved ability to write) if the posterior portion of the corpus callosum is involved.

Right Posterior Cerebral Artery Lesion

Occlusion of the right PCA results in a left-sided visual field defect and left-sided sensory loss if the thalamus is involved. There may also be associated neglect of the left side.

Vertebrobasilar Artery Infarction

Occlusion of a vertebral or basilar artery will present with either isolated or combined cerebellar and brainstem signs. These can include vertigo, diplopia, nystagmus, weakness or numbness in all four extremities or on one side of the body, ataxia, vomiting, occipital headache, or crossed motor or sensory findings.

For example, an infarction of the dorsal lateral medulla results in Wallenberg's syndrome. The lesion usually results from occlusion of the vertebral artery or one of its penetrating branches. The clinical symptoms and findings typically include ipsilateral ataxia, ipsilateral Horner's syndrome, and ipsilateral facial sensory loss with contralateral impairment of pain and temperature in the arm and leg (i.e., crossed sensory loss). Also, the patient typically has nystagmus and vertigo and may have hiccups or difficulty swallowing. There is no associated motor weakness because the corticospinal tracts travel anteriorly in the medulla and are spared.

Pure Motor Stroke

A pure motor stroke involving the face, arm, and leg on one side of the body that is fairly equal in severity in the affected body parts is caused by a lesion in the posterior limb of the internal capsule or base of the pons. There should not be associated impairment of higher cortical functions or sensory or visual loss.

Pure Sensory Stroke

A pure sensory stroke typically involves numbness of the face, arm, and leg on one side of the body and is usually caused by a lesion in the thalamus. There should not be associated weakness or impairment of higher cortical functions or visual loss.

DIAGNOSTIC STUDIES

Once the diagnosis of stroke is made, one considers diagnostic tests to confirm the diagnosis and exclude other possible causes for the neurologic deficits, such as tumor or brain abscess, and to clarify the underlying cardiovascular or hematologic cause. Therapeutic op-

1. Caplan LR. Caplan's Stroke: A clinical approach. Third edition. Boston. Butterworth–Heinemann, 2000: p. 67

tions are highly dependent upon the etiology of the stroke. Therefore, the evaluation of patients with brain ischemia includes brain and vascular imaging studies and routine blood work (i.e., complete blood count; serum electrolytes including glucose, serum cholesterol, and lipids; and other tests as warranted by the history) to confirm the diagnosis and to help differentiate an ischemic or hemorrhagic etiology.

Computed tomographic (CT) scans of the head are good for identifying hemorrhagic strokes because blood appears hyperdense (Fig. 14–5); they are also useful for identifying ischemic strokes, which appear hypodense (Fig. 14–6). CT scans, however, are somewhat limited in identifying acute ischemic strokes, because they are often not visualized until 12 to 24 hours after the onset of symptoms. Also, CT scans are not as sensitive at identifying strokes in the brainstem or cerebellum because of artifact from surrounding bone.

Magnetic resonance imaging (MRI) of the head, especially with diffusion-weighted imaging (DWI), is especially sensitive for identifying acute ischemic strokes, with the area of infarction demonstrating an area of restricted diffusion that appears bright on MRI scans. The MRI scan is also sensitive for detecting infarcts in the brainstem or cerebellum. Additionally, with susceptibility sequences, the MRI can reliably identify cerebral hemorrhages which appear hypointense.

If an ischemic stroke is identified, one must consider whether the cause is an embolus or thrombus. In the case of hypoperfusion, a history of myocardial infarction with significantly reduced cardiac output or hypotension is usually apparent. The location of thrombus or source of embolus can be investigated noninvasively with magnetic resonance angiography (MRA) or CT angiography of the head and neck, which can visualize stenotic lesions in the internal carotid artery or in the vessels of the circle of Willis. Doppler ultrasonography is another noninvasive method of investigating for carotid stenosis, and transcranial Doppler ultrasound (TCD) can be used to look for the presence of intracranial stenosis and to monitor for emboli passing under the probe.

Other tests include echocardiography to assess for the possibility of a thrombus in the heart or an atrial septal defect allowing for a paradoxical embolus. The electrocardiogram (ECG) can assess the possibility of a myocardial infarction causing the stroke and rule out atrial fibrillation, which is associated with an increased risk of embolism.

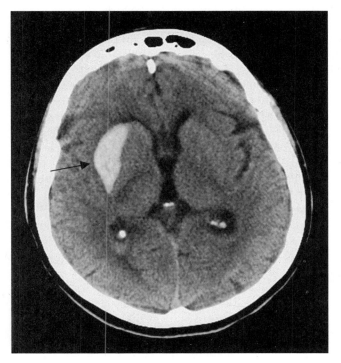

Figure 14–5 Computed tomographic scan of the head showing a hyperdense focal hemorrhage in the right basal ganglia, which is a common location for hypertensive hemorrhages. (Reproduced with permission from Bkushan V, Le T, Amin C, Nguyen H, Sharma N. Underground clinical vignettes: neurology. Malden, MA: Blackwell Science, 1999:17.)

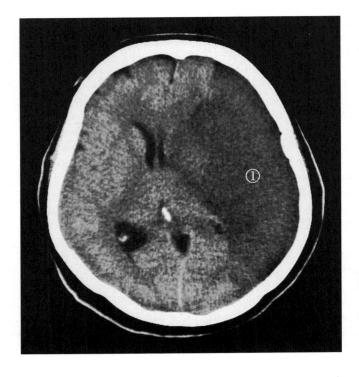

Figure 14–6 Computed tomographic scan of the head showing a large hypodensity (1) that represents a complete left middle cerebral artery infarct. (Reproduced with permission from Bkushan V, Le T, Amin C, Nguyen H, Sharma N. Underground clinical vignettes: neurology. Malden, MA: Blackwell Science, 1999:19.)

The tests discussed above are aimed at confirming the diagnosis and establishing a mechanism of injury. The etiology of the stroke may also be suggested by the neurologic findings. For example, pure sensory and motor strokes are typically caused by small lacunar strokes in the thalamus and internal capsule, respectively. Lacunar strokes are thought to be caused by occlusion of small penetrating arteries through a process called *lipohyalinosis* caused by chronic hypertension. Microatheromas can also obstruct penetrating arteries, causing branch infarcts and lacunes.

◆ KEY POINTS ◆

1. Wallenberg's syndrome results from occlusion of the vertebral artery.

2. Most lacunar strokes are caused by lipohyalinosis and microatheroma.

TREATMENT

Treatment is targeted at the underlying pathophysiologic process. For example, patients with greater than 70% stenosis of the carotid artery on the side responsible for TIAs or a stroke should be considered for carotid endarterectomy. This has been shown to decrease the risk of future ipsilateral strokes. If there is no evidence for carotid artery stenosis, then antiplatelet agents such as aspirin, clopidogrel, or dipyridamole are commonly used. Anticoagulation with heparin (acute treatment) or warfarin (long term) is considered if there is evidence for atrial fibrillation or another cardiac source of embolism. However, the benefit of anticoagulation must be weighed against the risk of hemorrhagic complications. Therefore, treatment must be considered on an individual basis.

Patients with acute ischemic strokes who present to the hospital within 3 hours of symptom onset may be candidates for thrombolysis with intravenous administration of recombinant tissue plasminogen activator (rt-PA). Because there is a significant risk for hemorrhage with rt-PA, there are strict exclusion criteria aimed at decreasing this risk.

Additionally, treatment for patients with ischemic stroke is aimed at maintaining adequate perfusion to the hypoperfused areas of brain at risk of infarction. These measures can include using isotonic intravenous fluids and maintaining an adequate blood pressure for brain perfusion.

For patients with hemorrhagic strokes, treatment depends on the underlying reason for hemorrhage. If the hemorrhage is due to an aneurysm, treatment is aimed at surgical repair, with either embolization or clipping of the aneurysm. On the other hand, if the hemorrhage is due to an underlying tumor, treatment will be tailored to investigating the type of neoplasm. The appropriate treatment may be surgical excision, chemotherapy, or irradiation, depending on the individual tumor type.

With acute hemorrhage, the coagulation profile (prothrombin time and partial thromboplastin time) should be checked, and fresh frozen plasma or vitamin K can be administered to correct bleeding abnormalities. Any anticoagulants or antiplatelet agents should be discontinued. Surgical decompression should be considered, especially for individuals with large superficial hemorrhages in the cerebral white matter or cerebellum. Chronic management includes treatment of hypertension and lifestyle modification to reduce stroke risk factors.

◆ KEY POINTS ◆

1. Treatment should be tailored to the individual patient based on the diagnostic evaluation for the underlying etiology.

2. Treatment options for ischemic stroke include rt-PA if the patient presents soon after symptom onset.

3. Treatment options include antiplatelet agents.

4. Anticoagulation with heparin or warfarin should be considered for patients with a cardiac source of embolism.

5. Hemorrhagic strokes should be evaluated to determine if an underlying lesion such as aneurysm or tumor is present.

15 Seizures

Seizures are among the most common problems in neurology. Up to 10% of the population will have a seizure at some point in their lives. In addition, seizures can be among the most dramatic forms of nervous system dysfunction. Although seizures have many different causes and manifestations, by definition a seizure is an abnormal hypersynchronous electrical discharge of neurons. Epilepsy is defined as a condition in which there is a tendency toward recurrent unprovoked seizures. Practically, the diagnosis of epilepsy is often applied after a patient has had two unprovoked seizures.

CLASSIFICATION OF SEIZURES

Seizures can arise from one portion of the brain (*partial*) or from the entire brain at once (*generalized*). Those that arise from one portion of the brain can evolve and spread to involve the whole brain (*secondarily generalized*). Among partial seizures, those in which awareness is impaired are termed *complex*, whereas those in which awareness is preserved are termed *simple*.

Simple Partial Seizures

By definition simple partial seizures begin in a focal area of the brain and do not impair awareness. In general, such seizures lead to positive rather than negative neurologic symptoms (e.g., tingling rather than numbness, hallucinations rather than blindness). The manifestations of simple partial seizures depend on their site of origin in the brain. Focal motor seizures, in which one part of the body may stiffen or jerk rhythmically, stem from the motor cortex in the frontal lobe. The classic Jacksonian march occurs when the electrical discharge spreads along the motor strip, leading to rhythmic twitching that spreads along body parts following the organization of the motor homunculus. Simple partial seizures from other regions of the brain can cause sensory phenomena (parietal), visual phenomena (occipital), or gustatory, olfactory, and psychic phenomena (temporal). The latter may include déjà vu, jamais vu, or sensations of depersonalization ("out of body") or derealization.

Complex Partial Seizures

Complex partial seizures have a focal onset and involve an impairment of awareness. They commonly arise from the temporal lobe, although some may originate in the frontal lobe as well. Complex partial seizures may include automatisms (stereotyped motor actions without clear purpose) such as lip-smacking, chewing movements, or picking at clothing. The patient may have speech arrest, or may speak in a nonsensical manner. By definition the patient does not respond normally to the environment or to questions or commands. Occasionally the patient may continue the activity she was participating in at the onset of the seizure, sometimes to remarkable lengths: Patients may continue folding the laundry during a seizure, or even finish driving home. Complex partial seizures of frontal lobe origin may involve bizarre bilateral movements, such as bicycling or kicking, or behavior such as running in circles.

Generalized Tonic-Clonic Seizures

Generalized tonic-clonic (GTC) seizures were formerly called *grand mal* seizures and are the seizure type with which the lay public is most familiar. They typically begin with a tonic phase, lasting several seconds, in which the entire body becomes stiff (including the pharyngeal muscles, sometimes leading to a vocalization known as the epileptic cry). This is followed by the clonic phase, in which the extremities jerk rhythmically, more or less symmetrically, typically for less than 1 to 2 minutes. Toward the end of the clonic phase the frequency of the jerking may peter out until the body finally becomes flaccid. The patient may bite his tongue and become incontinent of urine during a GTC seizure. There is typically a postictal state after the seizure, lasting minutes to hours, during which the patient may be tired or confused, before returning slowly back to normal.

Absence Seizure

An absence seizure is a generalized seizure that most commonly occurs in children and is characterized primarily by an unresponsive period of staring lasting several seconds, with immediate recovery afterward. Absence seizures can occur tens or even hundreds of times a day, and may first be diagnosed by schoolteachers as daydreaming or difficulty concentrating. A classic 3-Hz spike-and-wave electroencephalographic (EEG) pattern accompanies absence seizures (Fig. 15–1). Hyperventilation is a common trigger.

Other Seizure Types

Rarer seizure types include atonic, tonic, and myoclonic seizures, all of which are generalized in onset.

◆ KEY POINTS ◆

1. A seizure is an abnormal hypersynchronous electrical discharge involving neurons in the brain.

2. Epilepsy is a tendency to experience recurrent unprovoked seizures.

3. Seizures may manifest with motor, sensory, or psychic phenomena and are usually character-

ized by positive rather than negative neurologic symptoms.

4. Partial seizures originate in a focal area of the brain but may become secondarily generalized; awareness is preserved during simple partial seizures and impaired during complex partial seizures.

5. Generalized seizures originate in the entire brain at once; tonic-clonic and absence seizures are examples of such seizures.

EPIDEMIOLOGY AND ETIOLOGIES

Seizures often have their onset in the very young and the very old (Fig. 15–2). Etiologies vary depending on age of onset. In infants, a variety of neonatal infections, hypoxic-ischemic insults, and genetic syndromes are common causes of seizures.

Febrile seizures are a special case. They are the most common cause of seizures in children, affecting up to 3% to 9% of this age group. They occur between 6 months and 5 years of age in the setting of a febrile illness without evidence of intracranial infection, and are usually generalized in onset. The risk of future epilepsy is very small unless the seizures are prolonged or partial in onset, or if other neurologic abnormalities or a family history of epilepsy is present.

Older children may also develop seizures related to head injury or meningitis; genetic syndromes continue to be a significant etiology in this age group. Among young adults, head injury and alcohol are common causes of new-onset seizures, but brain tumors become one of the most common etiologies by middle age. Finally, in the elderly, strokes become the most common etiology, and metabolic disturbances from systemic problems such as hepatic or renal failure are a frequent cause as well.

Frequently, seizures occur in children (and sometimes adults) as part of a syndrome that may include specific seizure types, EEG patterns, and associated neurologic abnormalities. The diagnosis of a specific syndrome may have implications both for genetic testing and for the proper choice of pharmacologic treatments. Examples of epilepsy syndromes are outlined in Table 15–1.

EEG TRACINGS

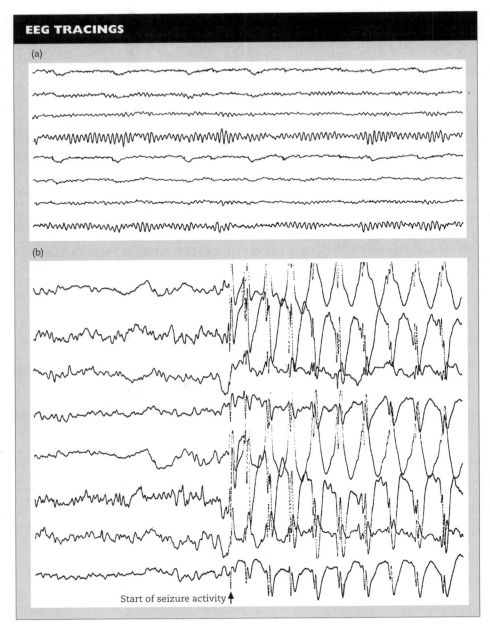

Figure 15–1   Characteristic EEG finding in absence seizures.
(a)   This tracing demonstrates a normal EEG recording of an awake adult. The top four channels are derived from electrodes over the left side of the head, from front to back, while the bottom four are derived from the right side of the head. A normal sinusoidal alpha rhythm is seen most prominently over the posterior head regions bilaterally (4th and 8th channels).
(b)   Midway through this tracing, rhythmic 3 Hz generalized spike-and-slow-wave discharges appear. This is the typical EEG pattern of an absence seizure; during these discharges, the patient may stare and be unresponsive. (Reproduced with permission from Ginsberg L. Lecture notes on neurology, 7th ed. Malden, MA; Blackwell Science, 1999:83.)

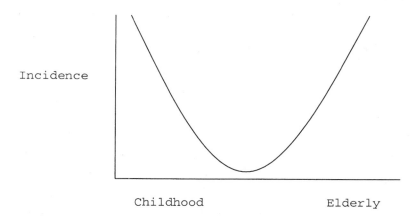

Figure 15–2 Incidence of new-onset seizures by age.

TABLE 15–1

Selected Epilepsy Syndromes

	Age of Onset	Seizure Types	Associated Findings	EEG Findings	Treatment
Lennox-Gastaut syndrome	Childhood	Tonic, atonic, myoclonic, generalized tonic-clonic, absence	Mental retardation	Slow (1–2 Hz) spike-and-wave	Valproic acid, lamotrigine, felbamate
Benign rolandic epilepsy	Childhood	Simple partial involving mouth and face, generalized tonic-clonic	Nocturnal preponderance of seizures	Centrotemporal spikes	Carbamazepine, no treatment
Absence epilepsy	Childhood and adolescence	Absence, generalized tonic-clonic	Hyperventilation as trigger	3-Hz spike-and-wave	Ethosuximide, valproic acid
Juvenile myoclonic epilepsy	Adolescence and young adulthood	Myoclonic, absence, generalized tonic-clonic	Early morning preponderance of seizures	4- to 6-Hz polyspike-and-wave	Valproic acid, lamotrigine

---

◆ **KEY POINTS** ◆

1. The incidence of new-onset seizures is highest among the very young and the very old.
2. Common etiologies of new-onset seizures differ depending on age of onset.
3. Febrile seizures in children are common and generally carry a benign prognosis.
4. Seizures may occur as part of specific epilepsy syndromes, characterized by distinctive seizure types, EEG patterns, or associated neurologic abnormalities.

DIAGNOSIS

Patient History

The diagnosis of seizures is a clinical one. Most commonly the patient will be seen after an event has occurred and the diagnosis will have to be made on the history alone. In these cases the patient (and more importantly, witnesses, if the seizure was not simple partial) must be pressed for an exact description of the event itself, any premonitory symptoms, and the character of the recovery period in order for the clinician to decide whether the event was a seizure and, if so, what type of seizure it was. It is these clinical details that should allow for the differentiation of seizures from other paroxysmal neurologic events (Table 15–2).

Physical Examination

Examination will be of diagnostic benefit in the rare instances in which the patient is seen while in the midst of the event or shortly thereafter. In the latter case a postictal hemiparesis, or Todd's paralysis, may be detected after a secondarily generalized seizure. Such a finding indicates that the seizure was of partial onset, even if that was not apparent to onlookers at the time. Other abnormalities on neurologic exam may also suggest the presence of a focal brain lesion. Of course, the general physical exam may yield findings suggestive of infection or other systemic disease that might explain a new-onset seizure. In particular, signs of meningitis should be sought in any patient who has had a seizure.

Laboratory Studies

Laboratory testing may reveal an underlying metabolic abnormality that might explain a new-onset seizure, such as hyponatremia or hypocalcemia. There is commonly a lactic acidosis, resulting in decreased serum bicarbonate, after a GTC seizure. In cases where infection is suspected, a lumbar puncture should always be performed.

Radiographic Imaging

An uncomplicated seizure in a patient with known epilepsy does not generally warrant head imaging. However, neuroimaging should usually be performed in

---

TABLE 15–2

Characteristics of Partial Seizures and Other Paroxysmal Neurologic Events

	Partial Seizures	Transient Ischemic Attacks (TIAs)	Migraines
Onset	Progression of symptoms over seconds	Sudden onset of symptoms	Progression of symptoms over 15–20 minutes
Neurologic symptoms	Positive motor or sensory symptoms, "psychic" symptoms such as déjà vu	Negative motor, sensory, or visual symptoms	Positive sensory or especially visual symptoms, such as scintillating scotomata
Duration	Usually less than a few minutes	Usually less than 30 minutes, always less than 24 hours	Symptoms for 15–20 minutes, followed by headache for up to hours
Consciousness	Impaired (if complex)	Preserved	Preserved
Headache	Occasionally postictal	None	Throbbing pain following progression of symptoms
Recovery	Postictal confusion, sleepiness	Immediate	Fatigue common
Risk factors	Structural brain lesion, family history of seizures	Hypertension, hyperlipidemia, smoking, diabetes	Family history of migraines

patients with new-onset seizures, with rare exceptions. For seizures of probable partial onset, an MRI is typically a necessary part of the diagnostic workup, to look for a structural abnormality that may serve as a focus for a partial seizure. A head CT may suffice in the urgent setting, however.

Electroencephalography

An EEG may be useful for several reasons: It may identify a potential focus of seizure onset, it may reveal characteristic findings that are diagnostic of a specific epilepsy syndrome, and it may establish whether a patient who has had a seizure and is still not waking up is merely postictal or is having continuous nonconvulsive seizures. However, the diagnosis of whether a particular paroxysmal event was a seizure or not must rest primarily on clinical grounds, because up to 50% of EEGs performed on known epilepsy patients may be normal.

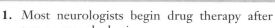

◆ KEY POINTS ◆

1. The diagnosis of seizures is a clinical one, and usually rests primarily on the history.

2. Certain elements of the history may help to differentiate seizures from other paroxysmal events.

3. Physical exam, laboratory studies, and neuroimaging may help to identify the cause of a new-onset seizure.

4. EEG may help to refine the diagnosis of seizures in particular settings.

TREATMENT

Drugs

The mainstay of epilepsy treatment is medical therapy. The number of available antiepileptic drugs (AEDs) has more than doubled in recent years, and there is now a large selection of agents from which to choose each with its own set of indications and adverse effects, (Table 15–3).

An AED is typically not started after a single seizure. This especially applies to symptomatic seizures, namely, those that are secondary to a treatable or reversible condition, such as meningitis, alcohol withdrawal, or hyponatremia. Most neurologists would also not start an AED after a single seizure for which no underlying cause is found.

AED treatment is usually begun after two seizures that are not symptomatic or provoked. The primary goal of AED usage is monotherapy—that is, control of seizures using a single drug. Most neurologists increase the dosage of a single drug until either seizure control is achieved or adverse effects become intolerable. If the latter occurs, the dose is lowered and a second drug added if necessary. If seizure control is achieved, an attempt is then made to taper the first drug, leaving the second as monotherapy. For about 70% of epilepsy patients, seizures will be well controlled on monotherapy. For the remainder, two or more AEDs may be required, or seizures may remain refractory to all medical therapy.

◆ KEY POINTS ◆

1. Most neurologists begin drug therapy after two unprovoked seizures.

2. Each drug has its own set of indications and adverse effects.

3. Monotherapy is the primary goal of antiepileptic therapy; most patients' seizures are well controlled on one medication.

Vagus Nerve Stimulation

The vagus nerve stimulator is a novel treatment device available in recent years that has been shown to be effective in the treatment of partial seizures. The device is implanted subcutaneously in the chest and stimulates the left vagus nerve through programmed electrical impulses delivered through leads placed in the neck.

Surgery

Patients refractory to medical management may be treated with epilepsy surgery. The most common surgical procedure is resection of the epileptogenic area, typically following a presurgical evaluation in which continuous video-EEG monitoring combined with neuroimaging and other tests is used to identify the focus of seizure onset. For seizures of medial temporal lobe origin, the rate of seizure freedom following resective

TABLE 15–3

Selected Antiepileptic Drugs

	Site of Action	Seizure Types Treated	Typical Adult Dosages	Characteristic Side Effects
Phenytoin (Dilantin)	Na^+ channel	Partial, generalized	300–500 mg/day	Gingival hyperplasia, coarsening of facial features
Carbamazepine (Tegretol)	Na^+ channel	Partial, generalized	600–2000 mg/day	SIADH, agranulocytosis
Valproic acid (Depakote)	Na^+ channel, GABA receptor	Partial, generalized, absence	1500–3000 mg/day	GI symptoms, tremor, weight gain, hair loss, hepatotoxicity, thrombocytopenia
Phenobarbital	GABA receptor	Partial, generalized	90–150 mg/day	Sedation
Ethosuximide (Zarontin)	T-type Ca^{++} channel	Absence	15–40 mg/kg/day (child)	GI symptoms
Gabapentin (Neurontin)	Unknown	Partial	1800–3600 mg/day	Sedation, ataxia
Lamotrigine (Lamictal)	Na^+ channel, glutamate receptor	Partial, generalized	300–500 mg/day	Rash, Stevens-Johnson syndrome
Topiramate (Topamax)	Unknown	Partial, generalized	200–400 mg/day	Word-finding difficulty, renal stones, weight loss
Tiagabine (Gabitril)	GABA reuptake	Partial	32–56 mg/day	Sedation

SIADH, syndrome of inappropriate secretion of antidiuretic hormone; GABA, γ-aminobutyric acid.

surgery may be as high as 90%. Other, less commonly used surgical procedures include corpus callosotomy, hemispherectomy, or multiple subpial transection.

STATUS EPILEPTICUS

Status epilepticus (SE) refers to an abnormal state in which either seizure activity is continuous for a prolonged period or seizures are so frequent that there is no recovery of consciousness in between them. There are several types of SE, including the generalized convulsive form (ongoing clonic movements of the extremities) and more subtle forms in which the patient may appear merely comatose or have subtle motor signs such as eyelid twitching or nystagmus. Potential etiologies of SE include acute metabolic disturbances, toxic or infectious insults, hypoxic-ischemic damage to the brain, and underlying epilepsy. Morbidity from SE can be high, and outcome depends largely on etiology and duration. SE is a medical emergency, and management centers on stopping the seizure activity and preventing the occurrence of systemic complications (Fig. 15–3).

SPECIAL TOPICS

First Aid for Seizures

All physicians should be familiar with first aid measures for those having a seizure. In general, the goal

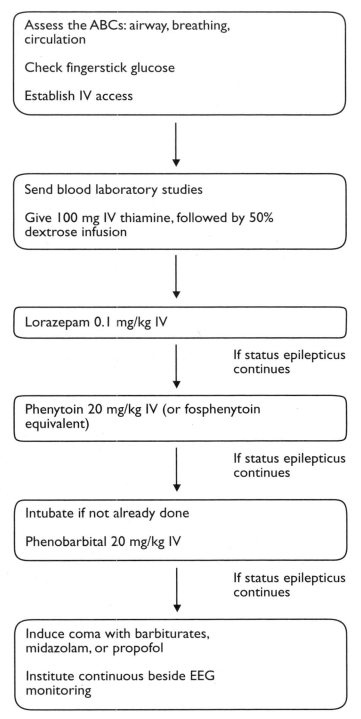

Figure 15–3 Neurologic emergency: status epilepticus.

is to prevent the patient from becoming injured and to prevent well-meaning bystanders from intervening unwisely. For complex partial seizures, the patient may wander or make semipurposeful movements; if necessary, she should be gently guided out of harm's way. More aggressive attempts at restraint may provoke a violent reaction. For GTC seizures, the patient should be laid on his side, if possible, so that vomiting does not lead to aspiration. Tight clothing should be loosened. *Nothing should be placed in the mouth.* Most GTC seizures stop within 1 to 2 minutes; immediate medical attention should be sought if one becomes more prolonged.

Seizures and Driving

Each state has its own licensing requirements for those with epilepsy, and physicians who care for seizure patients should be aware of these. Most states require a specific seizure-free interval before a patient may drive; exceptions can sometimes be made for purely nocturnal seizures or those with a prolonged simple partial onset that provides the patient with a warning without impaired awareness. A few states require physicians to report patients with seizures to the department of motor vehicles.

Antiepileptic Drugs and Pregnancy

Women taking AEDs have a somewhat higher risk of fetal malformations than the general population, though the absolute risk is still low. Valproic acid specifically has been associated with a higher rate of neural tube defects. All women with epilepsy who are considering becoming pregnant should take folic acid (1 mg or more per day). It is reasonable to consider modifying a woman's AED regimen prior to conception depending on the severity of her epilepsy, but the risk of anticonvulsant teratogenicity must be balanced with the risk of seizure occurrence during pregnancy.

Psychogenic Nonepileptic Seizures

A reported 10% to 30% of patients evaluated at tertiary referral centers for medically refractory epilepsy actually have events resembling seizures that have no EEG correlate and are felt to be psychogenic in nature. Some of these patients may also have true epileptic seizures at other times. Many patients with psychogenic events have comorbid psychiatric illnesses or a history of abuse in their past. Continuous video-EEG monitoring to record the typical events may be the most reliable method of differentiating psychogenic events from epileptic seizures.

Movement Disorders

IDIOPATHIC PARKINSON'S DISEASE

Idiopathic Parkinson's disease (PD) is a chronic degenerative disorder with characteristic clinical findings, response to L-dopa replacement therapy, and pathological changes in the brain. *Parkinsonism* is a term used to describe a heterogeneous group of conditions that share some of the clinical features of idiopathic PD but differ partially in their clinical expression, response to L-dopa therapy, and their underlying pathological substrates.

Epidemiology

PD is a common neurodegenerative condition. Most instances are sporadic, although there are reports of familial PD in which mutations in the α-synuclein and parkin genes have been described.

Pathology

PD is characterized by the progressive death of selected neuronal populations, notably the ventral tier of the neuromelanin-containing dopaminergic neurons of the substantia nigra pars compacta. The pathological hallmark of PD is the Lewy body.

Clinical Features

The four cardinal clinical features of idiopathic PD are tremor, rigidity, bradykinesia, and postural instability. Features that may be useful in distinguishing idiopathic PD from other parkinsonian syndromes are summarized in Table 16–1.

The tremor is slow (3–5 Hz) and most prominent when the limb is at rest. It affects the distal arm more often than the leg and is described as "pill rolling." It may also affect the lips, chin, and tongue. Rigidity typically affects the distal limbs more than the axial musculature and is described as "lead pipe" or "cogwheel." Slowness of movement (bradykinesia) and thought (bradyphrenia) are common features in idiopathic PD. Postural instability is the result of impaired postural reflexes and is largely responsible for falls. Dementia is increasingly recognized as an important feature of PD and occurs in 25% to 30% of patients as the disease advances.

Treatment

Replacement of the deficient dopamine with its precursor L-dopa is the mainstay of treatment. L-Dopa is administered because dopamine does not cross the blood-brain barrier. It is given together with a peripheral decarboxylase inhibitor (e.g., carbidopa) in a combined formulation (e.g., Sinemet). Carbidopa prevents the peripheral conversion of L-dopa to dopamine and thus reduces the incidence of peripheral dopaminergic side effects such as nausea, vomiting, and hypertension.

Dopaminergic agonists have been proposed as an alternative initial agent for symptomatic treatment, but the evidence that early therapy with dopaminergic agonists (e.g., ropinirole) may reduce the subsequent risk of dopa-induced dyskinesias, is controversial.

TABLE 16–1

Parkinsonian Syndromes

Parkinsonian Syndrome	Distinguishing Clinical Features
Progressive supranuclear palsy	Supranuclear ophthalmoplegia, with limitation of vertical more than horizontal gaze; axial rigidity and neck extension; early falls as a consequence of impaired postural reflexes, neck extension, and inability to look down
Corticobasal ganglionic degeneration	Apraxia, cortical sensory impairment and alien-limb phenomenon; severe unilateral rigidity; stimulus-sensitive myoclonus
Diffuse Lewy body disease	Early dementia; prominent visual hallucinations; extreme sensitivity to extrapyramidal side effects of antidopaminergic neuroleptic drugs
Vascular parkinsonism	"Lower-half" parkinsonism with rigidity in the legs and marked gait impairment; other evidence of diffuse vascular disease (corticospinal tract dysfunction, pseudobulbar palsy)
Multiple system atrophy	Early and prominent features of autonomic dysfunction; evidence of corticospinal tract dysfunction; cerebellar signs; stimulus-sensitive myoclonus; vocal cord paresis

A number of other agents have been used in early PD. The anticholinergics may be particularly useful in the treatment of tremor-predominant disease. Amantadine may be helpful for the early treatment of bradykinesia, rigidity, and gait disturbance. The selective mono-amine oxidase B inhibitor selegiline may also provide early symptomatic benefit. The catechol-O-methyl transferase inhibitors are the most recent addition to the antiparkinsonian armamentarium. They decrease removal of L-dopa and thereby augment its effects.

There has been a recent resurgence in lesioning and deep brain stimulation for the treatment of PD. These procedures target the motor thalamus, the internal segment of the globus pallidum, or the subthalamic nucleus.

◆ KEY POINTS ◆

1. Idiopathic PD results from loss of dopaminergic neurons in the substantia nigra.
2. The pathological hallmark is the Lewy body.
3. Tremor, rigidity, bradykinesia, and postural instability are the four cardinal symptoms.

DRUG-INDUCED MOVEMENT DISORDERS

Drugs with dopamine receptor blocking activity have a particular propensity for inducing a variety of movement disorders including akathisia, acute dystonic reactions, parkinsonism, tardive dyskinesia, and the neuroleptic malignant syndrome.

Neuroleptic malignant syndrome is an uncommon disorder characterized by muscular rigidity, fever, autonomic lability, altered level of consciousness, elevated creatine kinase level, and leukocytosis. Treatment involves discontinuation of the offending agent, antipyretics, rehydration, and occasionally the use of bromocriptine or dantrolene.

Akathisia is a dysphoric state characterized by the subjective desire to be in constant motion and is often associated with an inability to sit or stand still. Anticholinergics and β-blockers have been used with the most success in the treatment of this disorder.

Tardive dyskinesia is an orolinguomasticatory dyskinesia that occurs as the most common (late and persistent) movement disorder complicating neuroleptic use. Commonly observed are chewing movements, lip smacking, and rolling of the tongue inside the mouth and up against the inside of the cheek. The limbs and trunk may also be affected. A history of dopamine receptor blocking drug usage is essential to the diagnosis. The offending drug should be discontinued when possible; further therapeutic benefit may be obtained from dopamine depleting agents such as reserpine and tetrabenazine.

◆ **KEY POINTS** ◆

1. Antipsychotics (haloperidol as well as the newer atypical agents) are the most common cause of drug-induced movement disorders.
2. The propensity of a drug to cause these movement disorders is related to its D_2-receptor blocking activity.

STIFF MAN SYNDROME

Stiff man syndrome is a rare disorder characterized by fluctuating and progressive muscle rigidity with spasms. It may occur as an autoimmune or paraneoplastic process. Symptoms usually begin with stiffness of the axial and trunk muscles, with spread to the proximal limb muscles with time. Patients develop a lumbar hyperlordosis with restricted movements of the hip and spine that leads to the description of the gait as like that of a tin man. Superimposed on this background rigidity, they develop paroxysmal painful muscle spasms, often provoked by sudden movement or startle.

Diagnosis rests on the characteristic clinical profile and the demonstration of continuous motor unit activity, without evidence of neuromyotonia, pyramidal or extrapyramidal dysfunction, or structural spinal cord disease. Cerebrospinal fluid (CSF) is usually normal, and antibodies directed against glutamic acid decarboxylase (GAD) may be present.

Benzodiazepines and baclofen are the most useful antispasticity agents. The presence of anti-GAD antibodies and the occurrence of the stiff man syndrome as a paraneoplastic syndrome have led some to use immunosuppressive therapy (steroids, plasmapheresis, intravenous immunoglobulins), with varying success.

◆ **KEY POINTS** ◆

1. Stiff man syndrome is characterized by chronic axial muscle rigidity and stiffness with superimposed painful muscle spasms.
2. Stiff man syndrome may be associated with anti-GAD antibodies.

TREMOR

Tremor is an involuntary rhythmic oscillation of a body part (arm, leg, head, jaw, lips, or palate). Tremor is described as *resting* (present while the body part is not moving), *postural* (emerges during sustained maintenance of a posture), or *action* (appears during a voluntary movement). Action tremor may increase as the target is approached (*intention* tremor). Common causes of the various types of tremors are summarized in Table 16–2.

Essential tremor (ET) is a condition in which postural tremor is the only symptom. It may begin at any age, develops insidiously, and progresses gradually. A family history is common, but not invariable. ET almost always affects the hands, but may also affect the head, face, voice, trunk, or legs. It is almost always bilateral. Improvement of the tremor with small quantities of alcohol is a characteristic feature. Primidone and propranolol are of proven benefit in the treatment of ET.

TABLE 16–2

Tremor

Resting
   Idiopathic Parkinson's disease
   Other parkinsonian syndromes

Postural
   Essential tremor
   Physiological tremor
   Drugs (e.g., theophylline, β-agonists)
   Alcohol

Action
   Cerebellum and cerebellar outflow tract dysfunction (e.g., infarction, multiple sclerosis, tumor, Wilson's disease, drugs)

◆ **KEY POINTS** ◆

1. Tremor is an involuntary rhythmic oscillation of a body part.
2. Parkinson's disease causes a resting tremor.
3. Essential tremor is the most common cause of postural tremor.
4. Action or intention tremor suggests disease of the cerebellum or its connections.

CHOREA

Chorea is defined as involuntary, abrupt, and irregular movements that flow as if randomly from one body part to another. Patients are often unaware of even severe chorea. One of the earliest symptoms may be clumsiness or incoordination. Involvement of bulbar muscles may cause dysarthria and dysphagia. Chorea is usually accompanied by an inability to maintain a sustained muscle contraction (motor impersistence). Classic examples include an inability to keep the tongue protruded (serpentine tongue) and the inability to maintain a tight handgrip (milk-maid grip).

There are many causes of chorea, and it is impossible to determine the etiology based simply on the phenomenology of the abnormal movements. It is necessary to consider the age and relative acuity of onset, the presence or absence of a family history, the presence of associated symptoms, and the distribution of the movements. The different causes are summarized in Table 16–3.

For treatment, haloperidol has been used with greatest success.

◆ **KEY POINTS** ◆

1. Chorea comprises involuntary, abrupt, and irregular movements that flow randomly from one body part to another.
2. Huntington's disease, post-streptococcal infection, systemic lupus erythematosus, thyrotoxicosis, and pregnancy are among the more common causes of chorea.

TABLE 16–3

Chorea

Hereditary
  Huntington's disease
  Neuro-acanthosis
  Wilson's disease
Drugs
  Neuroleptics
  Antiparkinsonian medications
Toxins
  Alcohol
  Anoxia
  Carbon monoxide
Metabolic
  Hyperthyroidism
  Hyperglycemia and hypoglycemia
  Hepatocerebral degeneration
Pregnancy
Immunologic
  Systemic lupus erythematosus
  Post-streptococcal (Sydenham's chorea)
Vascular
  Caudate infarction or hemorrhage

BALLISM

Ballism is defined as large-amplitude and poorly patterned flinging or flailing movements of a limb that are frequently unilateral (*hemiballismus*). It usually results from a contralateral lesion in the caudate, putamen, or subthalamic nucleus. Stroke is the most common cause.

Dopamine depleting and blocking agents are the most useful treatment. When ballism is severe, contralateral thalamotomy or pallidotomy may be beneficial.

DYSTONIA

Dystonia is sustained muscle contraction leading to repetitive twisting movements or abnormal postures. The dystonias are classified as idiopathic or symptomatic. Recognition of secondary or symptomatic causes of dystonia is important because this may influence treatment.

A characteristic feature of dystonic movements is that they may be diminished by sensory tricks such as gently touching the affected body part (*geste antagoniste*). Dystonic movements tend to be exacerbated by fatigue, stress, and emotional states and may be suppressed by relaxation and sleep. Dystonia typically worsens during voluntary movement. At the time of onset, dystonia may only be present during a specific movement (action dystonia). With progression, however, the dystonia may emerge with other movements and eventually may be present at rest. Thus, dystonia at rest usually represents a more severe form than a pure action dystonia. Early onset of dystonia at rest should raise suspicion of an underlying (secondary) cause. Other clinical features that suggest that the dystonia is symptomatic include the presence of associated neurologic abnormalities or involvement of one side of the body only (hemidystonia).

Idiopathic torsion dystonia is a primary dystonia and may occur as a familial condition. The spectrum of the disorder is broad and includes focal (blepharospasm, torticollis, spasmodic dysphonia, writer's cramp), segmental, and generalized forms. The gene for the autosomal dominant familial form has been located on chromosome 9q, and mutations have been identified in the ATP-binding protein designated *A*.

Secondary causes of dystonia include metabolic disorders (e.g., Wilson's disease) degenerative diseases (Parkinson's disease, progressive supranuclear palsy, corticobasal ganglionic degeneration, Huntington's disease, multiple system atrophy), and nondegenerative central nervous system disorders (anoxia, head or peripheral trauma, prior stroke, multiple sclerosis, or drug-induced).

◆ KEY POINTS ◆

1. Dystonia is a sustained muscle contraction leading to repetitive twisting movements or abnormal postures.
2. Idiopathic torsion dystonia is a familial condition that may manifest as torticollis, writer's cramp, blepharospasm, or spasmodic dysphonia.

MYOCLONUS

Myoclonus is a sudden lightning-like movement produced by abrupt and brief muscle contraction (positive myoclonus) or inhibition (negative myoclonus or asterixis).

The four etiologic categories are essential, physiological, epileptic, and symptomatic. *Essential* myoclonus is a nonphysiological variety that occurs in isolation without evidence of other neurologic symptoms or signs. It may occur in familial and sporadic forms. Some patients may note a striking improvement with small quantities of alcohol. The causes of the other varieties of myoclonus are summarized in Table 16–4.

Clonazepam and valproate are used with greatest success in the management of myoclonus.

◆ KEY POINTS ◆

1. Myoclonus is a sudden lightning-like movement produced by abrupt and brief muscle contraction.
2. Clonazepam is the most effective treatment for many patients.

TICS

Tics are abrupt, stereotyped, coordinated movements or vocalizations. They may vary in intensity and be repeated at irregular intervals. The individual will frequently describe an inner urge to move, may be able to temporarily suppress the movement at the expense of mounting inner tension, and then obtain relief from the performance of the movement or vocalization. Tics may be exacerbated by stress and relieved by distraction.

Tics may be motor or vocal and are classified as being either simple or complex. Examples of simple motor tics include eye blinking, shoulder shrugging, and toe curling. Spitting and finger cracking are examples of complex motor tics. Simple vocal tics may take the form of sniffing, throat clearing, snorting, or coughing. The best recognized example of a complex vocal tic is coprolalia (involuntary obscene utterances). Tics may also be classified as idiopathic (the majority) or secondary. Secondary causes include head trauma, encephalitis, stroke, and various drugs.

TABLE 16–4

Myoclonus

Physiologic
  Hypnic jerks
  Anxiety and exercise induced
  Hiccups
Essential
Epileptic
  Primary generalized epilepsies (e.g., juvenile
    myoclonic epilepsy)
  Myoclonic epilepsies (often associated with
    encephalopathy or ataxia)
Symptomatic
  Metabolic encephalopathy (uremia, liver failure,
    hypercapnia)
  Wilson's disease
  Creutzfeldt-Jakob disease
  Hypoxic brain injury

Tourette's syndrome is a genetic disorder characterized by motor and vocal tics with onset in childhood. Boys are affected more than girls, although there is some suggestion that obsessive-compulsive disorder (OCD) may represent the phenotypic expression of the same genetic defect in girls. The motor and vocal tics may change over time. There is a trend toward periodic remission and exacerbation. In general, the disease is most active in adolescence and tends to diminish in severity during adulthood. There is an association with learning disability and OCD.

Pediatric autoimmune neurologic disorders associated with streptococcal infection (PANDAS) is a relatively recently described syndrome in which children develop exacerbation of tics and/or OCD following a group A β-hemolytic streptococcal infection. The proposed, although unproved, etiology is that the streptococcal infection triggers an autoantibody response that cross-reacts with components of the basal ganglia in susceptible individuals.

For treatment of tics, dopamine antagonists (haloperidol or the atypical antipsychotics) are most effective; however, because of the adverse effect profile of these agents, less potent drugs such as clonazepam and clonidine should be tried first.

◆ KEY POINTS ◆

1. Tics are abrupt, stereotyped, coordinated movements or vocalizations.
2. Tourette's syndrome is a common genetic disorder with onset of motor and vocal tics in childhood.
3. Dopamine antagonists are the most effective therapy for tics.

WILSON'S DISEASE

Wilson's disease (WD) is an autosomal recessive disorder of copper metabolism. The clinical presentation is usually with liver dysfunction and neuropsychiatric symptoms.

WD results from mutation of a copper-binding protein, dysfunction of which results in impaired conjugation of copper to ceruloplasmin and entry of copper into the biliary excretory pathway. This results in accumulation of copper within the liver and spillover into the systemic circulation with deposition in the kidney, cornea, and central nervous system.

Neurologic manifestations of WD include tremor, ataxia, dysarthria, dyskinesia, parkinsonism, and cognitive dysfunction, as well as disturbances of mood and personality. The Kayser-Fleischer ring is a golden brown or greenish discoloration in the limbic region of the cornea that results from copper deposition in Descemet's membrane. Kayser-Fleischer rings are almost invariably present in untreated patients with neurologic involvement.

In diagnosing WD, increased serum copper and decreased serum ceruloplasmin levels are expected, but not always present. Increased 24-hour urinary copper excretion is the most sensitive screening test. Diagnosis may be confirmed by demonstrating increased copper staining on liver biopsy.

Copper chelation with D-penicillamine has been the traditional therapy for WD. More recently, there has been a trend toward using a less toxic chelator, trientine, in conjunction with zinc. Therapy is lifelong. Given the inherited nature of this disorder, family members of an affected individual should be screened.

◆ KEY POINTS ◆

1. Wilson's disease is a disorder of copper metabolism.

2. Hyperkinetic and hypokinetic movement disorders, as well as cognitive, personality, and mood disturbances, are the most common neurologic manifestations of Wilson's disease.

3. Kayser-Fleischer rings represent copper deposition in the cornea.

4. Elevated serum copper levels, low ceruloplasmin levels, and elevated 24-hour urinary copper are useful screening tests.

PAROXYSMAL DYSKINESIAS

The paroxysmal dyskinesias are a rare group of movement disorders characterized by recurrent attacks of hyperkinesis with preserved consciousness. In paroxysmal kinesogenic choreoathetosis (PKC), episodes of chorea, athetosis, or dystonia are triggered by sudden movements and last for seconds to minutes. Attacks of paroxysmal (nonkinesogenic) dystonic choreoathetosis (PDC) are longer, lasting minutes to hours, and are triggered by alcohol, fatigue, and stress. In paroxysmal exercise-induced dystonia, episodes of dystonia are induced by sustained exercise and may persist for a number of hours. PKC is most effectively treated with agents such as carbamazepine.

17 Head Trauma

In the United States, trauma is the leading cause of mortality and morbidity for people aged 1 to 44 years. Head injury can result in seizures, permanent physical disability, or cognitive impairment. Furthermore, in more than half of trauma-related deaths, head injury is a significant contributor to mortality. There are approximately 500,000 new cases of traumatic brain injury per year in the United States, and these figures do not include the cases that do not come to medical attention. Of the 500,000 patients with traumatic brain injury, approximately 50,000 die before reaching the hospital. The rest are admitted; 80% of those have mild injury and 10% each have either moderate or severe injury.

Despite the serious nature of injury, mortality associated with severe head injury has decreased from 50% in the 1970s to 30% in the 1990s. The improvement is thought, in part, to be due to widespread use of computed tomographic (CT) scanners, establishment of trauma centers, better-trained medical personnel, and aggressive neurocritical care. In order to manage the patient with traumatic brain injury, it is important to be able to recognize the type of brain injury and to classify the severity of injury.

CLASSIFICATION

The most commonly used scale to classify the degree of severity of brain injury is the Glasgow Coma Scale (GCS) (Table 17–1). The GCS score is the sum of three scores (eye opening, best verbal response, and best motor response). The maximum score is 15; the minimum is 3. Head injury is classified as mild if the GCS score is 14 to 15, moderate if 9 to 13, and severe if 3 to 8. This classification combined with the type of cerebral injury helps to determine the prognosis.

INITIAL MANAGEMENT

As for all patients in the emergency ward, the initial assessment and management of a patient with traumatic brain injury focuses on airway protection, breathing, and circulation. Most patients with severe traumatic brain injury have damage to at least one other system. Thus, while the patient is being stabilized with respect to the respiratory and cardiovascular systems, a general medical examination should be conducted. Particular attention should be paid to signs of basal skull fracture, such as raccoon's eyes (periorbital ecchymoses), Battle's sign (postauricular ecchymoses), hemotympanum, or signs of cerebrospinal fluid leakage from the nose or ear. Initially, the neurologic examination should be focused on the level of consciousness as measured by the GCS, pupillary light reflexes, and extraocular movements. After the patient's cardiovascular status is stabilized, a more detailed neurologic examination should be performed.

TABLE 17–1

Glasgow Coma Scale

Points	Best Eye Opening	Best Verbal	Best Motor
6	—	—	Obeys commands
5	—	Oriented	Localizes pain
4	Spontaneous	Confused	Withdraws to pain
3	To speech	Inappropriate	Decorticate posturing
2	To pain	Incomprehensible	Decerebrate posturing
1	None	None	None

◆ KEY POINTS ◆

1. The Glasgow Coma Scale is used to classify the severity of traumatic brain injury.
2. Initial management is aimed at stabilizing the patient's respiratory and cardiovascular status.

TYPES OF BRAIN INJURY

After obtaining the history and performing an examination, all patients with a focal neurologic exam or who have a GCS score of less than 15 should have a head CT scan. A noncontrast CT scan of the head is particularly sensitive in detecting hemorrhage. Patients who are older than 14 years with a perfect GCS score of 15, no loss of consciousness, and a nonfocal neurologic examination can be discharged home without further testing provided that there is someone at home who can observe the patient for signs of deterioration.

For patients with a focal neurologic exam or a GCS score less than 15, the CT scan along with the neurologic exam will help determine the type and severity of injury to the brain. The major types of cerebral injuries are described below. Obvious lesions such as penetrating wounds from gunshot and stabbing have been excluded.

Acute Subdural Hematoma

Acute subdural hematoma (Fig. 17–1) is the most common focal intracerebral lesion in patients with severe brain injury, with an incidence of approximately 30%.

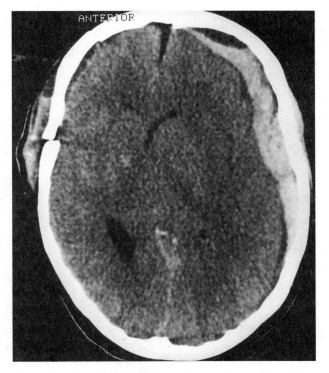

Figure 17–1 Typical CT scan appearance of a subdural hematoma with increased density on the left cerebral hemisphere. (Reproduced with permission from Ginsberg MD, Bogousslavsky J. Cerebrovascular disease: pathophysiology, diagnosis, and management. Malden, MA: Blackwell Science, 1998:1554.)

Tearing of the bridging veins between the cerebral cortex and the venous sinuses causes subdural hematomas and can occur spontaneously or with mild trauma, particularly in older people. Traumatic subdural hematomas are often associated with cerebral contusions, intracerebral hematomas, and brain lacerations. Acute subdural hematomas can be associated with high morbidity and mortality due to parenchymal damage underlying the hematoma and raised intracranial pressure caused by the additional volume occupied by the hematoma. Presentation can be varied and can include focal neurologic deficits, headache, or altered mental status.

Epidural Hematoma

In the majority of cases, epidural hematoma results from a skull fracture that lacerates the middle meningeal artery and causes accumulation of blood between the dura and the skull. The classic presentation of a patient with an epidural hematoma is brief loss of consciousness followed by a lucid interval for several hours and then change in the level of consciousness with hemiparesis on the side opposite the hematoma and ipsilateral pupillary dilation. On CT scan, epidural hematomas are hyperdense with a biconvex (lenticular) shape (Fig. 17–2). Mortality and morbidity are relatively low (5%–10%) provided the hematoma is diagnosed and treated with surgical drainage within a few hours.

Contusions

Contusions and intracerebral hematomas are a continuum and are high-density areas on head CT that represent bruises of the brain parenchyma. As such, they typically occur in areas where sudden deceleration of the head causes the brain to impact on bony prominences. Therefore, the majority of contusions occurs in the inferior frontal or temporal lobes. Contusions are sometimes described as *coup* (abnormalities seen directly below the site of impact) and *contrecoup* (abnormalities located on the opposite side of the brain as it is thrust against the skull). These patients are typically followed clinically and with follow-up head CT scans. Surgery is reserved for patients with significant mass effect and clinical deterioration.

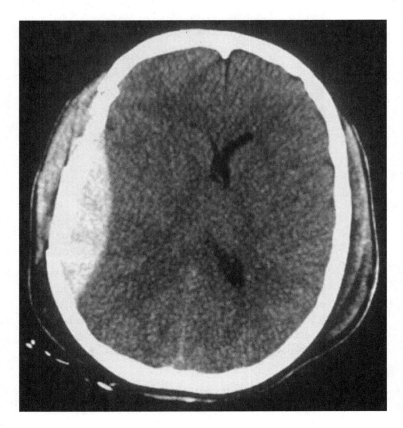

Figure 17–2   Head CT demonstrating the typical hyperdense lens-shaped appearance of an epidural hematoma. (Courtesy of David M. Dawson, M.D., Brigham & Women's Hospital.)

Subarachnoid Hemorrhage

Subarachnoid hemorrhage (SAH) is caused by bleeding into the subarachnoid space (Fig. 17–3) and is most commonly caused by trauma. In patients with traumatic brain injury, SAH is usually found in association with either contusions or hematomas. Management of patients with SAH involves monitoring for cerebral vasospasm, increased intracranial pressure, and acute hydrocephalus (for further discussion, see Chapter 14).

Diffuse Axonal Injury

Diffuse axonal injury or diffuse axonal shearing is a primary lesion caused by rotational acceleration and deceleration of the head. This is most commonly seen with patients who have been injured in motor vehicle accidents. It is also the most common presumed cause of coma in patients with head injury in the absence of a space-occupying lesion on head CT scan. Diffuse axonal injury is characterized by gross and microscopic axonal changes in the cerebral white matter and small hemorrhagic lesions of the corpus callosum and brainstem (Duret's hemorrhages).

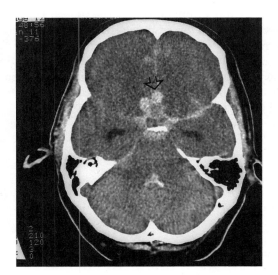

Figure 17–3 CT scan of the head showing subarachnoid hemorrhage characterized by hyperdensity in the subarachnoid space outlining the circle of Willis. (Reproduced with permission from Ginsberg MD, Bogousslavsky J. Cerebrovascular disease: pathophysiology, diagnosis, and management. Malden, MA: Blackwell Science, 1998:1260.)

HERNIATION SYNDROMES

The cranial cavity is essentially a closed space with a set volume that must contain the brain parenchyma, blood supply to the brain, and cerebrospinal fluid. If a mass lesion is present, either from tumor or blood, intracranial pressure will rise because the total volume is constant. The rise in intracranial pressure occurs after initial compensatory mechanisms, such as squeezing out of venous blood and cerebrospinal fluid, fail. Once intracranial pressure starts to rise, it does so in an exponential fashion. As intracranial pressure continues to rise, it results in distortion and displacement of the brain, which can in turn result in compression of critical brain structures, which gives rise to the following herniation syndromes.

Uncal (Tentorial) Herniation

Uncal herniation occurs with mass lesions of the middle cranial fossa. The uncus, the inferior medial portion of the temporal lobe, herniates downward into the posterior fossa between the rostral brainstem and the tentorium cerebelli. Typically, the third cranial nerve is entrapped, resulting in a unilateral dilated pupil. As the herniation progresses, hemiparesis and alteration of consciousness can occur, with eventual brainstem signs and changes in respiratory patterns. In the latter stages of herniation, death is imminent.

Cingulate Herniation

Cingulate herniation occurs when there is a mass lesion, usually in the frontal lobes, causing displacement of the cingulate gyrus across the falx cerebri. There are no specific signs or symptoms of this type of herniation, but it can frequently be seen on CT scan.

Central (Transtentorial) Herniation

Central herniation occurs when a large supratentorial mass causes downward displacement of the diencephalon and midbrain through the tentorial opening. Clinical findings include altered consciousness, bilateral small reactive pupils, and decorticate posturing followed by decerebrate posturing. Cheyne-Stokes respirations (crescendo-decrescendo pattern followed by a respiratory pause) can be seen. Cheyne-Stokes respirations are nonspecific and imply bilateral cerebral dysfunction from a variety of causes ranging from increased intracranial pressure to an underlying metabolic abnormality. In the terminal stage, tone is flaccid and respirations become slow and irregular.

Tonsillar Herniation

Tonsillar herniation occurs when a posterior fossa mass causes herniation of the cerebellar tonsils through the foramen magnum. The cerebellar tonsils compress the medulla, resulting in eventual respiratory arrest. Usually, tonsillar herniation is rapidly fatal.

◆ KEY POINTS ◆

1. The four major herniation syndromes are cingulate, uncal (tentorial), central (transtentorial), and tonsillar.

2. Uncal herniation is commonly recognized by a unilaterally dilating pupil.

3. Herniation is a medical emergency requiring prompt recognition and management.

MANAGEMENT

Once a patient is discovered to have a hemorrhage or herniation syndrome, neurology and neurosurgery consultations should be obtained for further management of the patient. It is beyond the scope of this chapter to discuss all the intricate management decisions in patients with brain injury. In addition to the initial management decisions of the patient with head injury described earlier in this chapter, if herniation or increased intracranial pressure is suspected, the patient must undergo urgent head CT. A large intraparenchymal hemorrhage or epidural hematoma will likely require surgical drainage. If suspicion for a herniation syndrome or increased intracranial pressure is high, the patient should be hyperventilated to achieve a P_{CO_2} between 25 and 30 mm Hg, which causes cerebral vasoconstriction and a rapid reduction of intracranial volume, which in turn decreases intracranial pressure. Additionally, mannitol (0.25–2.0 g/kg) can be administered. This is an osmotic diuretic that decreases intracranial volume and pressure temporarily. It must be remembered that these measures treat the symptom of increased intracranial pressure causing herniation but that the underlying cause may need to be treated in other ways.

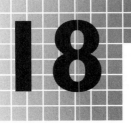

Systemic and Metabolic Disorders

The central and peripheral nervous system may be affected by a range of systemic and metabolic diseases. A few of these disorders have been selected for more detailed description in this chapter. Table 18–1 summarizes the more common neurologic manifestations of those systemic disorders that are not discussed below.

HEPATIC ENCEPHALOPATHY

Hepatic encephalopathy is a general term used to describe the altered mental state that accompanies liver failure. It encompasses two entities: the encephalopathy of fulminant hepatic failure and the portal-systemic encephalopathy that is associated with cirrhosis and portal hypertension or that may develop following portacaval shunting.

Clinical Presentation

The encephalopathy of fulminant hepatic failure progresses rapidly from mild inattention to stupor and coma within days. The essential feature of portal-systemic encephalopathy is the presence of waxing and waning cerebral dysfunction in the setting of liver failure. Traditionally, hepatic encephalopathy is graded in severity on a scale from 0 (normal) to 4 (coma). The intermediate stages are characterized by impaired attention and concentration, altered sleep patterns, abnormal visuospatial perception, and subtle personality changes.

Asterixis (negative myoclonus) is usually present. Other neurologic findings may include increased muscle tone, hyperreflexia, and extensor plantar responses.

Pathophysiology

The pathophysiology of hepatic encephalopathy is incompletely understood but is thought to result from the accumulation of neurotoxic substances (e.g., ammonia) that leads to increased brain glutamine concentrations, depressed glutamatergic neurotransmission, and increased expression of the peripheral-type benzodiazepine receptors. Manganese deposition in the basal ganglia may also play a pathogenic role.

Pathology

The Alzheimer type II astrocyte is the pathological hallmark of this disorder. These astrocytes appear to be metabolically hyperactive, and this has led to the suggestion that hepatic encephalopathy is a primary astrocytopathy.

Diagnosis

The diagnosis is usually suspected clinically on the basis of the encephalopathy in the context of liver failure. Hepatic synthetic function is impaired, with low serum albumin and prolonged prothrombin time (PT) and partial thromboplastin time (PTT). The electroencephalogram (EEG) may demonstrate triphasic waves, and magnetic resonance imaging (MRI) may reveal

---

TABLE 18–1

Neurologic Manifestations of Systemic Disease

Disease	Manifestations
Polyarteritis nodosa	Mononeuropathy multiplex, seizures, stroke
Churg-Strauss	Mononeuropathy multiplex, encephalopathy, stroke, chorea
Giant cell arteritis	Headache, blindness, polyneuropathy, stroke
Wegener's granulomatosis	Mononeuropathy multiplex, cranial neuropathy, basal meningitis
Rheumatoid arthritis	Myelopathy
Systemic lupus erythematosus	Affective or cognitive disorder, stroke, chorea, distal sensory polyneuropathy
Sjögren's syndrome	Sensory polyneuropathy
Behçet's disease	Aseptic meningoencephalitis
Cryoglobulinemia	Transient ischemic attack, stroke, peripheral neuropathy
Disseminated intravascular coagulation	Encephalopathy
Thrombotic thrombocytopenic purpura	Encephalopathy, seizures, stroke
Whipple's disease	Dementia, seizures, myoclonus, ataxia, supranuclear ophthalmoplegia, oculomasticatory myorhythmia

increased T1 signal in the basal ganglia, but these findings are not specific. In a patient with known liver disease who develops encephalopathy, it is important to identify underlying precipitating factors such as gastrointestinal hemorrhage, infection, increased dietary protein intake, drugs, constipation, or hypokalemia.

Treatment

Treatment should be directed toward the underlying cause of the liver disease when possible and to the alleviation of precipitating factors. Lactulose, titrated to produce two to three stools per day, is the mainstay of symptomatic therapy.

◆ KEY POINTS ◆

1. The essential feature of portal-systemic encephalopathy is the presence of waxing and waning cerebral dysfunction in the setting of liver failure.

2. Asterixis is frequently present.

3. Hepatic encephalopathy is thought to be a primary astrocytopathy.

4. Lactulose and the treatment of precipitating factors are the mainstay of therapy.

NEUROSARCOIDOSIS

Sarcoidosis is a multisystem granulomatous disorder of unknown etiology. Pulmonary disease is most common, and involvement of the nervous system occurs in around 5% of cases. It is very uncommon for sarcoidosis to involve the nervous system in the absence of other systemic disease.

Clinical Presentation

Sarcoidosis may involve almost any part of the central or peripheral nervous system. Cranial neuropathy due to chronic basal meningitis is the most common presentation of neurosarcoidosis, with the facial and optic nerves most frequently affected. Facial neuropathy may also occur due to parotid inflammation. Visual changes are common and may be due to direct involvement of the optic nerve, its meningeal covering, or uveitis. Raised intracranial pressure with papilledema may result from a space-occupying lesion, diffuse meningeal involvement, or hydrocephalus. Meningoencephalitis may manifest with cognitive and affective symptoms, and hypothalamic involvement may cause hypopituitarism, diabetes insipidus, sleep disturbance, obesity, and thermoregulatory disturbance. Space-occupying lesions may become apparent because of seizures or focal deficit. Myelopathy may result from an infiltrating or focal granulomatous process. Peripheral nerve involvement may manifest as a symmetric distal polyneuropathy or mononeuropathy multiplex.

Pathology

The typical pathology is that of noncaseating granulomata.

Diagnosis

Definitive diagnosis of neurosarcoidosis requires positive histology from affected tissue. Since there is often reluctance to obtain brain parenchymal or meningeal biopsy, the diagnosis is often presumptive, based on a consistent clinical presentation and histology from an alternative site. Cerebrospinal fluid (CSF) is frequently abnormal, with elevated protein and lymphocytic pleocytosis, but may be normal in the context of focal parenchymal disease. Serum angiotensin converting enzyme (ACE) concentration may be elevated. CSF ACE levels are often difficult to interpret in the context of elevated CSF protein. MRI may demonstrate white matter lesions, hydrocephalus, parenchymal mass lesion, nodular meningeal enhancement, or involvement of the optic nerve or spinal cord.

Treatment

Steroids are the mainstay of therapy. Although often used, there are limited data regarding the use of steroid-sparing agents such as methotrexate and azathioprine.

◆ KEY POINTS ◆

1. Sarcoidosis is a multisystem granulomatous disorder.

2. The nervous system is mostly affected in conjunction with systemic disease, but it may also be affected in isolation.

3. Cranial neuropathy and basal meningitis are common.

DIABETES MELLITUS

Diabetes mellitus is common in patients with neurologic disease, primarily because the nervous system is susceptible to the damaging effects of impaired glycemic control. However, there are also a number of disorders that are characterized by both diabetes and neurologic symptoms. These include mitochondrial diseases, myotonic dystrophy, Friedreich's ataxia, and the stiff man syndrome.

Peripheral neuropathy is the most common complication of diabetes mellitus and takes many forms (Table 18–2). Distal symmetric sensory polyneuropathy is the most common. Onset of this neuropathy is insidious, and it may often be asymptomatic. There is a predilection for involvement of small myelinated and unmyelinated fibers, with the result that loss of temperature and pinprick sensation are the most commonly reported symptoms. There may be associated distal motor neuro-

---

TABLE 18–2

Diabetic Neuropathies

Hyperglycemic neuropathy
Generalized neuropathies
    Distal symmetric predominantly sensory
      polyneuropathy
    Autonomic neuropathy
    Chronic inflammatory demyelinating
      polyradiculopathy (CIDP)
Focal neuropathies
    Cranial neuropathies (especially III, IV, and VI)
    Thoracolumbar radiculopathy
    Focal compression and entrapment neuropathies
    Proximal diabetic neuropathy (diabetic amyotrophy)
    Mononeuropathy multiplex

pathy, but it is invariably minor. Once established, this neuropathy is largely irreversible. The incidence of this complication is reduced in type 1 diabetic patients by strict glycemic control. There is frequently an associated autonomic neuropathy, the common symptoms of which include gustatory sweating, orthostatic hypotension, diarrhea, and impotence. Neurogenic bladder and gastroparesis occur less frequently.

Focal peripheral neuropathies also occur more commonly in diabetic patients. These include cranial neuropathies (most commonly cranial nerves III, IV, and VI) and focal compression neuropathies such as distal median neuropathies (carpal tunnel) and meralgia paresthetica (compression of the lateral cutaneous nerve of the thigh). Radiculopathy, especially truncal, occurs with greater frequency in diabetic patients. Typically, these radiculopathies manifest with nonradicular pain, truncal sensory loss, and focal weakness of the muscles of the anterior abdominal wall. Spontaneous recovery within a few months usually occurs.

The entity of proximal diabetic neuropathy is well recognized, but poorly understood. Another term that has been used to describe at least some of the patients with this disorder is *diabetic amyotrophy*. At least some of these proximal neuropathies are immune mediated, perhaps involving a vasculitis, and respond to treatment with steroids and other immunosuppressive therapies. Finally, chronic inflammatory demyelinating polyradiculopathy (CIDP) occurs more commonly in patients with diabetes.

Hyperglycemia may affect both the peripheral and the central nervous system. There is a syndrome of an acute distal sensory neuropathy that presents with dysesthesias and pain in the feet. This typically resolves with establishment of the euglycemic state. Nonketotic hyperglycemia (common in type 2 diabetes mellitus) may produce lethargy and drowsiness as well as focal or generalized seizures. An uncommon manifestation of nonketotic hyperglycemia is a syndrome of dystonia and chorea that is associated with reversible T1 signal hyperintensity in the basal ganglia. Finally, cerebral edema may complicate diabetic ketoacidosis. Children are particularly susceptible to this potentially fatal complication.

Many of the symptoms of hypoglycemia are referable to the nervous system, including headache, blurred vision, dysarthria, confusion, seizures, and coma. Repeated episodes of hypoglycemia may produce injury to the anterior horn cells of the spinal cord and result in a syndrome similar to amyotrophic lateral scle-

rosis. Recurrent and prolonged hypoglycemia may also lead to the development of permanent cognitive deficits.

Cerebrovascular disease (transient ischemic attacks and stroke) is more common in diabetic patients, with hypertension being the main risk factor for stroke among patients with diabetes. Most ischemic strokes in diabetic patients are due to intracranial small vessel disease (lacunar stroke).

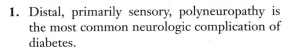

◆ KEY POINTS ◆

1. Distal, primarily sensory, polyneuropathy is the most common neurologic complication of diabetes.

2. Hyperglycemia may cause seizures, focal neurologic deficit, transient painful peripheral neuropathy, and occasionally chorea.

3. Stroke occurs more commonly in diabetic patients.

ALCOHOL AND NUTRITIONAL DISORDERS

Alcohol may adversely affect the nervous system in many ways (Table 18–3), and the manifestations of vitamin deficiency (Table 18–4) are frequently associated with alcoholism. Two of the better-known syndromes that result from alcohol abuse and vitamin deficiency are presented in more detail below.

Wernicke's Encephalopathy and Korsakoff's Syndrome

Wernicke's encephalopathy and Korsakoff's syndrome are related conditions that represent different stages of the same pathologic process. Wernicke's encephalopathy is characterized by the clinical triad of ophthalmoplegia, (truncal) ataxia, and confusion that develops over a period of days to weeks. Associated signs and symptoms include impaired pupillary light response, hypothermia, postural hypotension, and other evidence of nutritional deficiency. The syndrome results from a deficiency of thiamine and may be precipitated by the administration of intravenous glucose. It is a clinical diagnosis and warrants immediate therapy with intravenous thiamine. Untreated, the condition is progressive and the mortality is high. Following the administration of thiamine, the

TABLE 18–3

Effects of Alcohol on the Nervous System

Condition	Manifestations
Peripheral neuropathy	Distal sensorimotor axonal neuropathy; recovery with abstinence is slow and incomplete
Cerebellar degeneration	Gait ataxia greater than limb ataxia, dysarthria, no nystagmus
Tobacco-alcohol amblyopia	Insidious and painless loss of vision; centrocecal scotoma
Marchiafava-Bignami syndrome	Frontal-type dementia, seizures and pyramidal signs; focal demyelination and necrosis of corpus callosum
Acute intoxication	Impaired cognition, ataxia, dysarthria, nystagmus, diplopia
Acute withdrawal	Agitation, insomnia, tremulousness, hallucinations, seizures
Wernicke's encephalopathy	Confusion, ataxia, ophthalmoplegia
Korsakoff's syndrome	Isolated memory disturbance with confabulation

TABLE 18–4

Vitamin Deficiency Syndromes

Symptom	Deficient Vitamin
Confusion and encephalopathy	Thiamine, niacin
Dementia	Vitamin B_{12}, folate, niacin
Seizures	Pyridoxine, niacin
Ataxia	Vitamin E, niacin
Myelopathy	Vitamins B_{12} and E, niacin
Peripheral neuropathy	Thiamine, pyridoxine, vitamins B_{12} and E, niacin

tions reflect the pathology within the dorsal columns and the lateral corticospinal tracts. The presentation is usually with insidious onset of paresthesias in the hands and feet. With time, weakness and spasticity may develop in the legs. Frequently, there is an associated large-fiber peripheral neuropathy (also due to the B_{12} deficiency). Hematologic abnormalities (macrocytic anemia) are variably present. Normal serum B_{12} levels do not preclude the diagnosis, and it may be necessary to measure levels of serum homocysteine and methylmalonic acid, the precursors of B_{12} (which are elevated when B_{12} is deficient). Partial improvement with B_{12} replacement therapy may be expected. Since folate is a necessary component to the B_{12} synthetic pathway, its deficiency (theoretically) may cause the same deficits as B_{12} deficiency. Typically, however, the hematologic abnormalities occur in isolation.

ocular signs resolve within hours and the confusion over days to weeks. The gait ataxia may persist. Once the global confusion has receded, isolated memory deficits may persist (Korsakoff's syndrome).

Subacute Combined Degeneration of the Spinal Cord

Subacute combined degeneration of the spinal cord results from vitamin B_{12} deficiency and derives its name from the degeneration of the posterior and lateral white matter tracts of the spinal cord. The clinical manifesta-

◆ KEY POINTS ◆

1. Wernicke's encephalopathy is characterized by the triad of confusion, ataxia, and ophthalmoplegia.

2. Subacute combined degeneration of the cord refers to the damaging effects of vitamin B_{12} deficiency on the posterior and lateral columns of the spinal cord.

CENTRAL PONTINE MYELINOLYSIS

Central pontine myelinolysis is a rare demyelinating disorder that occurs most often in alcoholic patients and may be precipitated by too rapid correction of hyponatremia. As the name indicates, the pons is most commonly affected, but the basal ganglia, thalamus, and subcortical white matter may also be involved. The clinical presentation is with an acute confusional state, spastic quadriparesis, locked-in syndrome, dysarthria, and dysphagia.

ANTIPHOSPHOLIPID SYNDROME

The antiphospholipid syndrome (APS) describes a disorder in which venous or arterial thrombosis, recurrent fetal loss, and thrombocytopenia are associated with elevated titers of antibodies that are directed against phospholipids. The presence of these antibodies may be demonstrated by solid-phase immunoassay (e.g., anticardiolipin antibody) or by the in vitro prolongation of the partial thromboplastin time (lupus anticoagulant). The APS may occur in isolation (primary APS) or in association with an underlying autoimmune disorder, most commonly systemic lupus erythematosus (secondary APS). Involvement of the nervous system is not uncommon in the antiphospholipid syndrome.

Clinical Presentation

Although most thrombotic episodes in patients with antiphospholipid antibodies are venous, when thrombosis does occur in the arterial circulation, the brain is most commonly affected. Both small- and large-vessel stroke have been reported, and cardiac embolism may result in embolic stroke. Sneddon's syndrome refers to the association between cerebral ischemia and livedo reticularis.

Diagnosis

Antiphospholipid antibodies should be sought in young patients with stroke or in patients with otherwise unexplained stroke, especially if any of the other features of the antiphospholipid syndrome are present. Diagnosis requires the demonstration of high titer IgG antiphospholipid antibodies on two occasions at least 6 weeks apart.

Treatment

Long-term anticoagulation with warfarin to achieve an international normalized ratio (INR) of 3 to 4 is the recommended therapy.

TABLE 18–5

Neurologic Manifestations of Hypothyroidism

Mental state: Poor concentration and memory, dementia, psychosis, coma

Seizures

Headaches: Pseudotumor cerebri

Cranial nerves: Papilledema, ptosis, tonic pupil, trigeminal neuralgia, facial palsy, tinnitus, hearing loss

Cerebellar ataxia: Truncal and gait ataxia more than limb ataxia; dysarthria; nystagmus

Muscles: Cramps, pain, and stiffness; proximal more than distal; creatine kinase level may be markedly increased

Neuromuscular junction: Association with myasthenia gravis

Nerves: Entrapment neuropathy (e.g., carpal tunnel), axonal polyneuropathy (improves with thyroxine replacement); delayed relaxation of deep tendon reflexes

Sleep apnea: Obstructive and central

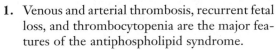

◆ **KEY POINTS** ◆

1. Venous and arterial thrombosis, recurrent fetal loss, and thrombocytopenia are the major features of the antiphospholipid syndrome.

2. Antiphospholipid antibody is a general term that encompasses the lupus anticoagulant, anticardiolipin antibodies, and antibodies directed against a mixture of various phospholipids.

3. Anticoagulation is the treatment of choice for antiphospholipid-associated stroke.

THYROID DISEASE AND THE NERVOUS SYSTEM

The nervous system is more commonly affected by hypothyroidism than by hyperthyroidism. Neurologic signs and symptoms are very rarely the only manifestations of thyroid disease. The periodic paralyses and proximal myopathy that are associated with the hyperthyroid state are discussed in Chapter 24. Seizures, chorea, and dysthyroid eye disease may also result from hyperthyroidism, and there is an association with myasthenia gravis. The range of neurologic manifestations of hypothyroidism is summarized in Table 18–5.

19 Brain Tumors

METASTATIC TUMORS

Metastatic brain tumors are more common than primary brain tumors. It is estimated that there are more than 100,000 new cases of metastatic brain tumors annually in the United States, compared with 16,800 new primary brain tumors in 1999. The most common metastatic intracranial tumor is from the lung, which accounts for almost half of the cases of metastases. Other common cancer types that metastasize to the brain are breast, melanoma, and renal cell carcinoma. Leptomeningeal metastases are most commonly caused by the acute leukemias, although lymphoma, breast, melanoma, and lung cancer can also be responsible. Dural-based metastases are caused by breast cancer, prostate, and lymphoma. However, the focus of this chapter will be on the primary brain tumors.

ETIOLOGY OF PRIMARY BRAIN TUMORS

r primary brain tumors is
cy between exposure and
0 years. Radiation of the
idence of tumors by up to
the tumor type. There is
lines, cell phones, and head
rain tumors. In most cases,
tumor is unknown.

CLINICAL MANIFESTATIONS

Patients with brain tumors can present with either generalized or focal signs. Generalized signs are usually due to increased intracranial pressure and consist of headache, papilledema, nausea, or vomiting. Headache is the presenting feature in 35% of patients and develops in up to 70% during the course of the disease. The headaches can be on the same side as the tumor but can also be generalized; they are typically worsened with Valsalva maneuvers that can increase intracranial pressure. Seizures are the presenting symptom in 15% to 95% of patients, depending on the tumor type. For example, seizures are more commonly associated with low-grade gliomas and meningiomas than other tumor types. The seizure can be either focal or generalized and may be associated with a postictal hemiparesis (Todd's paralysis) or aphasia. Other focal signs associated with primary brain tumors include progressive hemiparesis.

DIAGNOSIS

The test of choice for diagnosis of a brain tumor is a contrast-enhanced magnetic resonance imaging (MRI) scan. Computed tomography (CT) is sometimes used because it is more widely available, lower in cost, and will detect over 90% of brain tumors. However, CT can miss structural lesions in the posterior fossa and low-grade non-enhancing tumors. A normal contrast-enhanced MRI of the head virtually rules out brain tumor.

Lumbar puncture for routine cerebrospinal fluid analysis as well as cytology is sometimes performed to rule out meningeal involvement of metastatic tumors and as part of the evaluation for primary central nervous system lymphomas. However, if the patient has elevated intracranial pressure, lumbar puncture is associated with risk of herniation and should be avoided.

CLASSIFICATION OF PRIMARY BRAIN TUMORS

The major categories of primary brain tumors are derived from the cell types present in the central nervous system that give rise to the neoplasm. The World Health Organization has presented a histologic classification of tumors of the central nervous system (Table 19–1). Some of the major types of brain tumors will be discussed below and in Table 19–2.

Glial Tumors

Glial tumors are divided into two major groups: astrocytic and oligodendroglial. Both can be either low or high grade. Low-grade astrocytomas have a peak incidence in the third and fourth decade of life. New-onset seizure is the typical presentation, and MRI usually shows a non-enhancing lesion that is bright on T2-weighted images. If the tumor is in an area amenable to surgery, resection is usually performed. If resection is not possible due to proximity to critical brain structures or large tumor size, radiation therapy is the treatment of choice. Median survival of patients with low-grade astrocytomas is approximately 5 years, although the range is broad and some patients can survive more than 10 years. Patients who die early usually have progression of their disease to high-grade malignant glioma.

The malignant astrocytomas are the most common glial tumors, and glioblastoma multiforme represents over 80% of the malignant gliomas. Glioblastoma usually affects patients in the sixth or seventh decade of life. MRI typically shows irregular contrast enhancement of the tumor that is almost ringlike (Fig. 19–1). The tumor involves the white matter and can spread

TABLE 19–1

Histologic Classification of Tumors of the Central Nervous System

Tumors of neuroepithelial tissue
  Astrocytic tumors
    Astrocytoma
    Anaplastic astrocytoma
    Glioblastoma multiforme
    Pilocytic astrocytoma
  Oligodendroglial tumors
    Oligodendroglioma
    Anaplastic oligodendroglioma
  Ependymal tumors
    Ependymoma
    Anaplastic ependymoma
  Choroid-plexus tumors
    Choroid-plexus papilloma
    Choroid-plexus carcinoma
  Embryonal tumors
    Medulloblastoma
    Primitive neuroectodermal tumor

Meningeal tumors
  Meningioma
  Hemangioblastoma

Primary central nervous system lymphoma

Germ-cell tumors
  Germinoma
  Choriocarcinoma
  Teratoma

Tumors of the sellar region
  Pituitary adenoma
  Craniopharyngioma

Metastatic tumors

Abridged from the World Health Organization classification.

across the corpus callosum, involving the other cerebral hemisphere. There is often associated edema that can be severe enough to cause mass effect and herniation. Treatment involves surgical resection as the initial step. However, because the tumor is widely infiltrative, radiotherapy must be used as adjuvant treatment. There is some controversy as to the effectiveness of chemotherapy, but despite aggressive treatment, median survival is

TABLE 19–2

Common Primary Brain Tumors

Tumor	Typical Age of Presentation (yr)	Treatment	Median Survival (yr)
Glial tumors			
Astrocytomas			
Low-grade astrocytoma	30–40	Surgery or radiation	5–10
Glioblastoma multiforme	60–70	Surgery and radiation	1–2
Oligodendroglioma	30–40	Chemotherapy	10
Medulloblastoma	<15	Surgery and radiation	5–10
Meningioma	>50	Surgery	Benign tumor

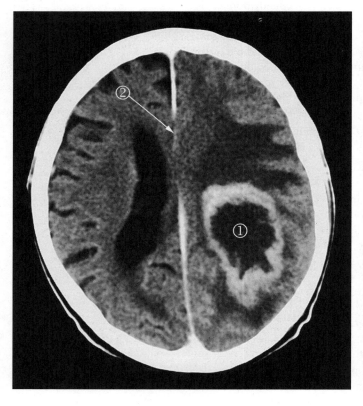

Figure 19–1   CT scan of the brain showing glioblastoma multiforme. Note the irregular enhancement pattern with contrast. There is also a central area of necrosis (1) with surrounding edema and mass effect (2). (Reproduced with permission from Bkushan V, Le T, Amin C, Nguyen H, Sharma N. Underground clinical vignettes: neurology. Malden, MA: Blackwell Science, 1999:45.)

approximately 1 year for patients with glioblastoma multiforme and up to 3 years for patients with other malignant astrocytomas such as anaplastic astrocytomas.

Oligodendroglial tumors are tumors derived from oligodendrocytes. Like astrocytomas, they can be either low or high grade (anaplastic), which is of both prog-nostic and therapeutic importance. These tumors are often difficult to distinguish radiologically from astrocytomas. Treatment, however, is different, with chemotherapy being the mainstay for both low- and high-grade oligodendrogliomas. Median survival is approximately 10 years.

Medulloblastoma

Epidemiology

Medulloblastoma is the most common malignant brain tumor of childhood and accounts for 25% of malignant primary brain tumors in children younger than 15 years.

Clinical Manifestations

The tumor arises from the cerebellum and therefore often presents with signs of increased intracranial pressure (headache, nausea, vomiting) when mass effect causes obstruction of the flow of cerebrospinal fluid in the aqueduct of the brainstem. Because the tumor usually arises from the midline of the cerebellum, neurologic findings include truncal ataxia and unsteadiness of gait.

Diagnosis

MRI or CT shows a contrast-enhancing tumor that is usually midline and often distorts or obliterates the fourth ventricle (Fig. 19–2). Medulloblastoma has a high tendency to metastasize to other parts of the central nervous system, so once the diagnosis is made, contrast-enhanced imaging of the entire brain and spinal cord is necessary. The tumor may also metastasize outside of the nervous system, particularly to bone. Therefore, a radionuclide bone scan and bone marrow aspirate should also be performed.

Treatment

Surgical resection is the first step in treatment. The goal is to remove as much tumor as possible without damaging the brainstem or causing permanent cranial nerve dysfunction. The next step is radiation therapy, and some centers also add chemotherapy. With treatment, the 5-year survival rate is approximately 50% to 75%, with the 10-year survival rate less than 50%.

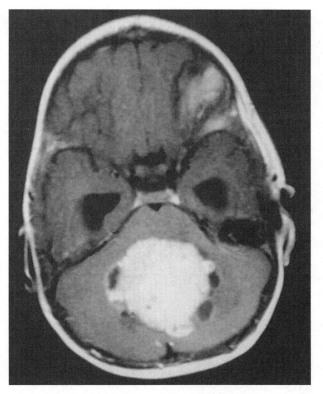

Figure 19–2 Medulloblastoma as shown by MRI scan with contrast enhancement. Note that the fourth ventricle and cerebral aqueduct are obliterated, resulting in hydrocephalus as shown by the enlarged ventricles in the temporal lobes. (Reproduced with permission from Black PM, Loeffler J. Cancer of the nervous system. Malden, MA: Blackwell Science, 1997:141.)

Meningioma

Meningiomas are the most common benign brain tumor and the second most common primary brain tumor after the gliomas. They represent approximately 20% of the intracranial neoplasms. Meningiomas are derived from the cells that form the outer lining of the arachnoid granulations of the brain. Thus, as the name implies, they are a meningeal-derived tumor, and strictly speaking, not a brain tumor.

Clinical Manifestations

Meningiomas can present with seizures, headaches, or focal neurologic deficits and are more common in women and tend to occur in later life. However, there are many patients with asymptomatic meningiomas that are discovered with neuroimaging for unrelated reasons. Over 90% of meningiomas are supratentorial and can involve the falx, cerebral convexities, sphenoid wing, or olfactory groove. Therefore, focal neurologic symptoms

vary depending on the brain structures compressed by the meningioma.

Diagnosis

Meningiomas can be diagnosed with either CT or MRI with contrast enhancement. On MRI, meningiomas can be missed with T1- and T2-weighted images, because they are isointense or slightly hyperintense. However, they are brightly enhancing with contrast (Fig. 19–3) and may show a "dural tail" at the margin of the tumor.

Treatment

Surgery is the primary treatment for meningiomas. However, asymptomatic meningiomas, especially those that are less than 2 cm in diameter without much associated edema, can be followed with annual CT scans with contrast. Even after complete resection, up to 20% recur within 10 years.

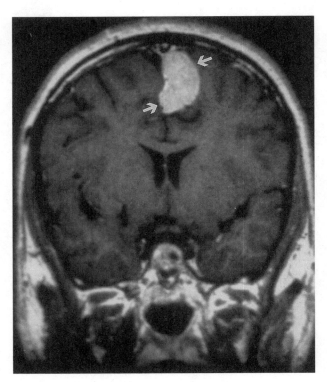

Figure 19–3 Coronal post-gadolinium MRI shows an enhancing parasagittal meningioma along the falx. (Reproduced with permission from Black PM, Loeffler J. Cancer of the nervous system. Malden, MA: Blackwell Science, 1997:68.)

◆ **KEY POINTS** ◆

1. Meningiomas are the most common benign brain tumor.
2. Treatment is surgical for symptomatic lesions and observation for small asymptomatic lesions.

Primary Central Nervous System Lymphoma

Primary central nervous system lymphoma (PCNSL) is a diffuse non-Hodgkin's lymphoma. Ninety-eight percent of PCNSLs are B-cell derived. PCNSL formerly represented less than 1% of all primary brain tumors. However, over the last two decades the reported incidence has tripled because of better detection methods and increased rates of acquired immunosuppression, especially the acquired immunodeficiency syndrome (AIDS), which increases the risk for PCNSL. However, the incidence of PCNSL has also increased among immunocompetent hosts for unclear reasons.

Clinical Manifestations

The lesions are multifocal in approximately 40% of cases and are usually subcortical. The most common presenting symptoms are cognitive and behavioral changes, but hemiparesis, aphasia, or seizures can also occur. In immunocompetent hosts, the peak incidence is in the sixth and seventh decades of life.

Diagnosis

Diagnosis is made with MRI that shows the lymphoma to be located periventricularly with diffuse and homogenous enhancement. Stereotactic biopsy is usually required for definitive diagnosis. PCNSL can disseminate to the cerebrospinal fluid in 25% of patients and to the eye in 20% of patients. Thus, lumbar puncture for cytology and formal ophthalmologic evaluation must be performed.

Treatment

Unlike for other primary brain tumors, surgery plays no role in the treatment of PCNSL. Treatment is with chemotherapy, usually methotrexate, which can penetrate the blood-brain barrier. Chemotherapy is often combined with irradiation, with a median survival of 3.5 years.

◆ KEY POINTS ◆

1. PCNSL has increased in frequency largely due to the increased number of patients with acquired immunodeficiency syndrome.
2. PCNSL can spread to the cerebrospinal fluid, eye, and bone.
3. PCNSL commonly presents with a change in mental status.
4. Treatment is chemotherapy with or without radiation.

Acoustic Neuroma

Strictly speaking, acoustic neuroma is not a primary brain tumor—it is a benign tumor of the eighth cranial nerve. It originates from the Schwann cell–glial cell junction of the vestibular portion of the nerve, so some authors have preferred calling the tumor *acoustic schwannoma* or *vestibular schwannoma*. These tumors account for 8% of all intracranial tumors and over 80% of all cerebellopontine angle tumors in adults. The tumors are typically unilateral, except in cases of neurofibromatosis type 2, where they can be bilateral.

Clinical Manifestations

The most common symptom is unilateral hearing loss. Other symptoms include unilateral tinnitus or other cranial nerve dysfunction, if the tumor becomes large enough to compress nearby cranial nerves.

Diagnosis

Audiometry is the best test for asymmetric unilateral sensorineural hearing loss. If imaging is warranted, MRI with contrast enhancement should be performed because the lesion enhances brightly with gadolinium.

Treatment

Because acoustic neuromas grow slowly, treatment options include observation, radiation therapy, and surgery. If the tumor is large, intervention should be considered because there is a risk for brainstem compression or hydrocephalus if the tumor continues to grow. Intervention should also be considered in patients with good hearing because delay in treatment may result in hearing impairment.

◆ KEY POINTS ◆

1. Acoustic neuroma is a benign tumor.
2. It presents typically with unilateral hearing loss.
3. Acoustic neuroma can be bilateral in neurofibromatosis type 2.

Pituitary Adenoma

Pituitary adenomas are the most common pituitary tumors. They can present with either neurologic or endocrine manifestations. Neurologically, the most common symptom is headache, and if the tumor continues to grow it can compress the optic chiasm located above the pituitary gland. This can result in bitemporal hemianopia because of the way that the visual fibers cross in the optic chiasm (see Chapter 4).

Endocrine manifestations are either hypofunction or hyperfunction. The most common endocrine manifestation of pituitary adenoma is hypopituitarism, especially of the gonadotropin and growth hormone systems. Hyperfunction of the pituitary gland can result in oversecretion of prolactin, causing galactorrhea; growth hormone excess, causing either acromegaly or gigantism; or excess corticotropin, causing Cushing's disease.

Surgery through a transsphenoidal approach is usually the initial treatment. Also, in patients with prolactin-secreting adenomas, dopamine receptor agonists such as bromocriptine are used.

20

Demyelinating Diseases of the Central Nervous System

MULTIPLE SCLEROSIS

Central nervous system (CNS) demyelinating diseases are characterized by the pathologic hallmark of acquired loss of myelin with relative preservation of axons. The most common and most well known of the CNS demyelinating diseases is multiple sclerosis (MS). For many reasons MS is also one of the most feared diagnoses in neurology: It strikes young healthy people in the prime of their lives, its course is marked by unpredictable relapses, almost any aspect of neurologic function may be affected, and the specter of lifelong disability requiring a wheelchair is a devastating one.

However, MS has a wide range of presentations and an equally wide range of prognoses, and effective treatments aimed at both the underlying disease process and some specific complications are available. For the student, the study of demyelinating diseases provides an excellent opportunity to learn about dysfunction of different parts of the CNS and to master the wide variety of neurologic exam abnormalities that accompany these disorders.

Epidemiology

MS is a chronic neurologic disease that begins most commonly in young adulthood. The peak incidence of MS is between 20 and 30 years of age. Women are affected twice as much as men. Its prevalence in the northern United States is about 60 per 100,000. As discussed below, there are epidemiologic patterns to suggest both environmental and genetic influences.

Geographically, MS is more common in northern latitudes. The incidence in Scandinavian countries is higher than that in Italy, and the incidence in the northern United States is higher than that in the South. However, there are racial differences as well (with a higher prevalence in white populations), and the implication of the geographic disparities is unclear. Interestingly, those who move from a low-risk to a high-risk geographic region or vice versa before the age of 15 adopt the risk of MS associated with their new home, while those who migrate after 15 retain the risk associated with their childhood home. This supports the theory that a latent viral infection acquired in childhood may play a role in the pathogenesis of the disease.

There is strong evidence supporting a genetic predisposition to MS as well. For example, there is an increased incidence of MS in monozygotic twins compared with dizygotic twins, as well as an increased incidence in association with particular HLA alleles.

Clinical Features

The classic neurologist's definition of MS is a disease marked by multiple lesions separated in space and time. This means that multiple distinct areas of the CNS must be involved (rather than one area recurrently, for example), and that the disease must not be just a monophasic illness (with multiple areas affected only once simultaneously, for example).

The clinical features are defined, as might be expected, by the location of the lesions. Thus, a right occipital lesion could result in a left homonymous hemianopia, while a right cervical spinal cord lesion may lead to an ipsilateral hemiparesis and loss of joint position sense with contralateral loss of pain and temperature sensation. Almost any neurologic symptom, in fact, can be produced by an MS lesion, depending on location.

Common clinical features (Table 20–1) include corticospinal tract signs such as weakness and spasticity, cerebellar problems such as intention tremor and ataxia, sensory abnormalities such as paresthesias and loss of vibration and proprioception, and bladder dysfunction. In later stages cognitive and behavioral abnormalities and seizures may occur. A few particular syndromes characteristic of MS warrant further description.

Optic neuritis (ON) is a common initial presenting symptom of MS. (This fact reminds us that the optic nerve is actually an extension of the CNS rather than a true peripheral nerve.) ON is characterized by a painful loss of visual acuity in one eye. The vision may be blurry and there may be loss of color discrimination; severe episodes may lead to actual blindness. Pain may be predominant when the eye moves (i.e., when looking around). On exam there is loss of acuity and color vision, and the optic disc may be swollen, with indistinct margins (papilledema). A past history of ON is suggested by the presence of red desaturation (subtle loss

TABLE 20–1	
Common Clinical Features of Multiple Sclerosis	
Neurologic System	*Clinical Sign or Symptom*

Cranial nerves	Optic nerve dysfunction
	  Visual acuity loss
	  Red desaturation
	  Papilledema or optic disc pallor
	  Relative afferent pupillary defect
	Eye movement disorders
	  Internuclear ophthalmoplegia
	  Nystagmus

Motor system	Weakness
	Spasticity
	Reflex abnormalities
	  Increased muscle stretch reflexes
	  Babinski signs
	  Clonus

Sensory system	Paresthesias Vibratory loss Joint position sense loss Lhermitte's sign
Cerebellar function	Ataxia Intention tremor Dysarthria
Autonomic system	Bladder dysfunction
Other	Fatigue Depression Uhthoff's phenomenon

of color appreciation), optic disc pallor or atrophy, and a relative afferent pupillary defect (RAPD).

Transverse myelitis describes an area of inflammatory demyelination in the spinal cord. Most commonly this is a partial lesion and does not mimic a complete spinal cord transection; rather, particular tracts may be interrupted at the level of the lesion in a patchy way. Thus, there may be unilateral or bilateral weakness or sensory loss below the lesion. Bowel and bladder function may be lost. Reflexes may be exaggerated below the lesion, and Babinski signs may be present. Patients may report a band of tingling or pain around the torso at the level of the lesion.

Internuclear ophthalmoplegia (INO) is not a common finding in MS patients, but it is quite characteristic. The presence of an INO in a young person suggests few other diagnostic possibilities. An INO results from dysfunction of the medial longitudinal fasciculus (MLF) and leads to an inability to adduct one eye when looking toward the opposite side, with associated nystagmus of the abducting eye. Adduction of both eyes when observing a near target (convergence) is preserved.

Other clinical features characteristic of MS include *Lhermitte's sign*, a tingling, electric sensation down the spine when the patient flexes the neck, and a worsening of symptoms and signs in the heat, a condition termed *Uhthoff's phenomenon.*

◆ KEY POINTS ◆

1. MS is characterized by multiple lesions separated in space and time.

2. Almost any neurologic symptom can occur, depending on the location and burden of lesions.

3. Features characteristic of MS include optic neuritis, transverse myelitis, internuclear ophthalmoplegia, Lhermitte's sign, and a worsening of symptoms in the heat.

Clinical Course and Prognosis

The majority of MS patients begins with a relapsing-remitting course (Fig. 20–1), in which there are discrete episodes of neurologic dysfunction (relapses or "flares") which resolve after a period of time (usually weeks to months). Unfortunately, such a course usually evolves into one in which recovery from each relapse is incomplete and baseline functioning deteriorates (secondary progressive). Rarely, patients may have a relentlessly progressive course from the onset, either with superimposed relapses (progressive-relapsing) or without (primary progressive).

To put the prognosis in broad terms, about one-third of MS patients lead lives of minimal disability and con-

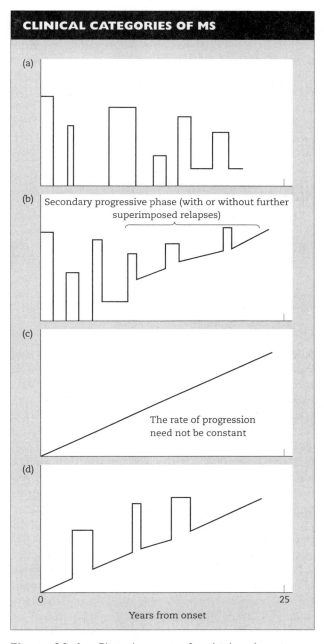

CLINICAL CATEGORIES OF MS

(a)

(b) Secondary progressive phase (with or without further superimposed relapses)

(c) The rate of progression need not be constant

(d)

0   Years from onset   25

Figure 20–1 Clinical course of multiple sclerosis: (a) relapsing-remitting, (b) secondary progressive, (c) primary progressive, (d) progressive-relapsing. (Reproduced with permission from Ginsberg L. Lecture notes on neurology, 7th ed. Malden, MA: Blackwell Science, 1999:141.)

tinue to work, about one-third have disability significant enough to prevent them from continuing at their jobs, and about one-third have severe disability, typically becoming wheelchair-bound. Features predicting a good prognosis include young age at onset, female sex, rapid remission of initial symptoms, mild relapses that leave little or no residual deficits, and a presentation with sensory symptoms or optic neuritis rather than motor symptoms.

◆ **KEY POINTS** ◆

1. Most MS patients have a relapsing-remitting course, which frequently evolves into a secondary progressive course.
2. Prognosis is quite variable and ranges from minimal to severe disability.

Diagnosis

The diagnosis of MS begins with a thorough history and examination. In particular, patients often present with what appears to be a single episode of neurologic dysfunction, but upon further questioning may recall past episodes of seemingly unrelated neurologic symptoms that may in fact represent prior lesions separated in space and time. It is important to inquire specifically about past neurologic symptoms, particularly those that suggest optic neuritis, transverse myelitis, or other typical MS features. On exam, as well, evidence of old optic neuritis or other neurologic lesions should be sought.

The two most useful laboratory studies are magnetic resonance imaging (MRI) and cerebrospinal fluid (CSF) analysis. On MRI, new MS lesions appear as discrete T2-hyperintense areas in the white matter of the brain or spinal cord. Fluid-attenuated inversion recovery (FLAIR) sequences also show these lesions particularly well (Fig. 20–2). Acute lesions may not be evident on T1-weighted images, but may enhance with gadolinium. Old, chronic MS lesions may become T1-hypointense, with a "black hole" appearance. MS lesions have a predilection for particular areas, including the periventricular white matter, the corpus callosum, and the cerebellar peduncles. Sagittal images may demonstrate foci of demyelination spreading upward from the corpus callosum, termed *Dawson's fingers*.

The characteristic CSF finding is oligoclonal bands,

found in more than 90% of MS patients at some point during their illness. These reflect intrathecal production of IgG antibodies by plasma cell clones. Although highly suggestive of MS, they can also be found in other neurologic disorders. Routine CSF studies during an acute relapse may show a mild pleocytosis and elevated protein. Calculation of the IgG index, based on relative levels of IgG and albumin in the CSF and serum, can also suggest intrathecal antibody production.

Finally, visual evoked potentials can be used in suspected MS to document evidence of old optic neuritis. There may be an increased latency of the P100 wave on the affected side.

◆ **KEY POINTS** ◆

1. The diagnosis of MS begins with a thorough history and examination, particularly directed toward identifying past episodes of neurologic dysfunction.
2. MRI is the best imaging modality to detect both new and old MS lesions.
3. The characteristic CSF abnormality is the presence of oligoclonal bands.
4. Visual evoked potentials may provide evidence of old optic neuritis.

Pathology

The histologic appearance of an acute MS lesion consists of a sharply defined area of myelin loss with relative preservation of axons, and associated signs of perivascular inflammation, including the presence of macrophages, lymphocytes, and plasma cells. Reactive astrocytes may be present.

Chronic MS lesions are hypocellular and have extensive glial proliferation.

Treatment

Treatment for MS falls into three categories: acute therapies for relapses, chronic therapies that treat the underlying disease process, and symptomatic therapies that address the various complications of the disease.

Acute relapses of MS are most commonly treated with corticosteroids. A course of IV methylprednisolone

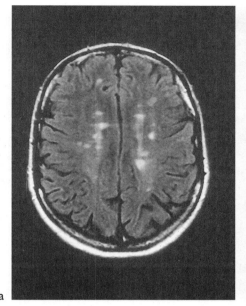

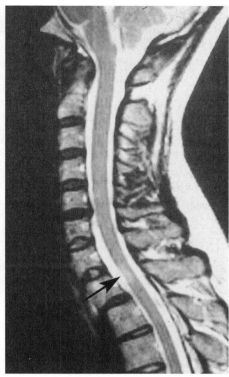

a

b

Figure 20–2 MRI images of multiple sclerosis lesions. (Reproduced with permission from Ginsberg L. Lecture notes on neurology, 7th ed. Malden, MA: Blackwell Science, 1999:142.)

followed by an oral prednisone taper is a common protocol. Although the effect of steroids on the long-term outcome is unclear, the duration of acute relapses is often shortened. A well-publicized trial demonstrated that IV steroids used to treat optic neuritis delayed but did not prevent the subsequent development of MS.

The therapies used in the chronic treatment of MS are immune-modulating agents (Table 20–2). These include beta-1a interferon and beta-1b interferon, which are available in injection form and have been shown to decrease the rate of relapses, the burden of lesions seen on MRI, and the rate of accumulated disability. Both are currently used in relapsing-remitting and some secondary progressive patients. Side effects can include flulike symptoms, depression, and injection site reactions; patients may develop neutralizing antibodies to the interferons that reduce their effectiveness. Glatiramer acetate is a polypeptide formulation injected

subcutaneously that is also used in relapsing-remitting patients.

In patients who no longer respond to the above therapies, other immunosuppressive agents may be used, including azathioprine, cyclophosphamide, or methotrexate. Mitoxantrone is a chemotherapeutic agent that may be useful. Of course, these agents have a wide range of accompanying toxicities.

Several of the symptomatic complications that accompany MS have specific treatments. Spasticity can be managed with baclofen, diazepam, or tizanidine. Bladder dysfunction can be managed with anticholinergic agents (for urinary urgency) as well as intermittent self-catheterization. Addressing urinary problems is particularly important to prevent recurrent infections that may trigger MS relapses and can lead to chronic renal disease. Unfortunately, there is no effective treatment for tremor or ataxia, which are common disabling symptoms.

TABLE 20–2

Immune-Modulating Agents Used in the Treatment of Multiple Sclerosis

Drug	Administration	Side Effects
Beta-1a interferon (Avonex)	30 mcg (6 million units) IM every week	Flulike symptoms, anemia, depression, development of neutralizing antibodies
Beta-1b interferon (Betaseron)	0.25 mg (8 million units) SQ every other day	Injection site reactions, flulike symptoms, depression, hematologic/liver abnormalities, development of neutralizing antibodies
Glatiramer acetate (Copaxone)	20 mg SQ every day	Injection site reactions, injection-related chest pain and shortness of breath

---

◆ KEY POINTS ◆

1. Acute MS relapses are treated with intravenous corticosteroids.

2. Interferons and glatiramer acetate are immune-modulating agents used to treat relapsing-remitting MS.

3. More toxic immunosuppressants are used in refractory cases.

4. Symptomatic therapies include those for spasticity and bladder dysfunction.

ACUTE DISSEMINATED ENCEPHALOMYELITIS

Acute disseminated encephalomyelitis (ADEM) is a monophasic illness leading to areas of demyelination within the CNS, commonly occurring following an antecedent viral infection or vaccination. ADEM may be difficult to distinguish from the initial presentation of MS.

Clinical and Radiologic Features

As in MS, almost any neurologic symptom or sign can occur, depending on the location of the demyelinating lesions. In ADEM, the lesions are multiple and are frequently more patchy, bilateral, and confluent than in MS, in which the lesions may be more discrete. ADEM lesions have a predilection for the posterior cerebral hemispheric white matter. Clinically, behavioral and cognitive abnormalities are often seen in ADEM, whereas they are uncommon until the late stages of MS. Radiologically, all areas of demyelination in ADEM appear acute and may enhance with gadolinium.

Diagnosis

The diagnosis of ADEM may be suspected based on the clinical presentation and radiologic findings. CSF typically will show a lymphocytic pleocytosis (with more cells than usually seen in MS) and an elevated protein. Oligoclonal bands are rarely present. When the illness is indistinguishable clinically or radiologically from the initial episode of MS, definitive diagnosis may not be possible unless or until a second episode of neurologic dysfunction occurs.

Prognosis and Treatment

By definition ADEM is a monophasic illness, and neurologic recovery is typically nearly complete. A course of IV corticosteroids is often administered to shorten the duration of the episode and lessen the severity of the symptoms.

21

Infections of the Nervous System

Infections of the nervous system are common and require urgent care. Therefore, it is important for clinicians to be able to recognize the common infections so that appropriate treatment can be initiated promptly. The major etiologic categories of infectious diseases are bacterial, viral, fungal, and parasitic.

BACTERIAL MENINGITIS

Bacterial meningitis results from the inflammatory response to infection of the leptomeninges. Bacteria can gain access to the central nervous system (CNS) by colonizing the mucous membranes of the nasopharynx with local tissue invasion. This leads to bacteremia and seeding of the subarachnoid space by hematogenous spread. Bacteria can also penetrate the subarachnoid space directly through skull or meningeal defects caused by trauma or surgery. Other potential sources are infections of parameningeal sites such as the ear, sinuses, and teeth (dental abscesses).

The most common symptoms of bacterial meningitis are fever, headache, confusion, and neck stiffness, but not all of the symptoms are always present. Diagnosis is made by lumbar puncture (LP) for cerebrospinal fluid (CSF) analysis. Especially if focal findings are present on exam, imaging of the brain with computed tomog-

raphy (CT) or MRI should be done to identify a brain abscess or other mass lesion. One should draw blood cultures and investigate for a primary source of infection. CSF examination typically reveals an elevated opening pressure (20–50 cm H_2O), elevated protein (100–500 mg/dL), decreased glucose concentration (<40% serum glucose), and pleocytosis (100–10,000 white blood cells per mL, normal <5) with a predominance of polymorphonuclear leukocytes. The CSF Gram stain is positive in 60% to 70% of the cases, with positive CSF cultures in 75% to 80% of cases.

Overall, the most common etiology of bacterial meningitis in adults is *Streptococcus pneumoniae*, which accounts for one-third to one-half of all cases (Table 21–1). Formerly, the most common cause of bacterial meningitis in children, was *Haemophilus influenzae*. However, since the widespread introduction of vaccination against *H. influenzae* type B, there has been an 82% reduction in *H. influenzae* meningitis in children. *S. pneumoniae* and *Neisseria meningitidis* are now the most common causes for bacterial meningitis in children older than 1 month.

Treatment depends on the LP results and local antibiotic resistance patterns. If the LP and Gram stain are nondiagnostic or if LP is delayed, empiric antibiotic therapy should be started. Empiric antibiotic treatment is aimed at treating the most common pathogens for a

TABLE 21–1

Common Etiologic Agents in Bacterial Meningitis

Age or Clinical Setting	Etiology	Empiric Treatment
Birth to 3 months	E. coli, group B streptococcus, L. monocytogenes	Ampicillin and broad-spectrum cephalosporin
3 months to 18 years	H. influenzae, N. meningitidis, and S. pneumoniae	Broad-spectrum cephalosporin*
18–50 years	S. pneumoniae and N. meningitidis	Broad-spectrum cephalosporin*
>50 years	S. pneumoniae, L. monocytogenes, and gram-negative rods	Ampicillin and broad-spectrum cephalosporin*
Head trauma or neurosurgical procedure	Staphylococci and gram-negative rods	Vancomycin and ceftazidime

*Add vancomycin if resistant pneumococcus is a significant local problem.

particular age group (see Table 21–1). Furthermore, the history and physical exam can help identify a particular pathogen. For example, *N. meningitidis* can be associated with a petechial rash and can be responsible for epidemics in crowded living areas such as those encountered by military recruits. Once the results from Gram stain or cultures are known, antibiotic coverage can be tailored using antibiotics that have high penetrance into the cerebrospinal fluid. Corticosteroids are used as adjunctive treatment in children and have been shown to decrease the incidence of hearing loss and other neurologic sequelae. There are no data to support the use of corticosteroids in adults with bacterial meningitis.

◆ KEY POINTS ◆

1. *S. pneumoniae* is the most common cause of bacterial meningitis in adults.
2. *N. meningitidis* can be responsible for epidemic meningitis in crowded conditions.

TUBERCULOSIS

Although tuberculosis (TB) is relatively uncommon in the United States, it is common in developing countries, with an incidence 15 times greater than in the United States. Approximately 1% of TB cases have a neurologic manifestation such as meningitis, a tuberculoma in the brain, or involvement of the spine (Pott's disease). TB meningitis is usually subacute to chronic in presentation but can begin acutely. In addition to the typical signs of meningitis, TB meningitis can present with cranial nerve palsies because inflammation and exudates often affect the base of the brain where the cranial nerves exit the brainstem. Hydrocephalus is another complication of basilar meningitis. In addition, if the inflammation affects blood vessels, patients can develop brain infarcts.

Diagnosis is made by identifying the tubercle bacillus on CSF acid-fast bacilli (AFB) smear or culture. Most patients have extrameningeal tuberculosis, so chest x-ray can be helpful, although pulmonary involvement is not invariable. Purified protein derivative testing (PPD) is positive in 50% of affected patients; it can be helpful if positive but does not exclude the disease if negative. CT or magnetic resonance imaging (MRI) with contrast enhancement can be helpful in demonstrating a tuberculoma in the brain or basilar inflammation characterized by enhancement of the basal meninges after contrast infusion. Spinal fluid analysis typically shows an elevated protein, low glucose, and lymphocytic pleocytosis. Spinal fluid cultures can take 6 to 8 weeks to return and can be negative in one-third of the cases. Thus, multiple spinal taps may be necessary and if suspicion is high enough, empiric treatment should be started.

Treatment for TB meningitis should involve isoniazid, rifampin, and pyrazinamide in order to avoid drug resistance. In severe cases with focal neurologic deficits, corticosteroids are added.

BRAIN ABSCESS

Brain abscess is caused by focal infection of the brain parenchyma itself. Abscesses usually arise from local spread of an infected contiguous site, such as the ear or sinuses, or hematogenous spread, especially from the lung. These abscesses tend to be solitary. If multiple brain abscesses are present, the cause is usually hematogenous spread from endocarditis or an immunocompromised state.

Patients with brain abscess typically present with signs of a space-occupying lesion. Fever, neck stiffness, and an elevated peripheral white count are not common features of brain abscess, in contrast to the signs and symptoms of meningitis. Diagnosis is made by MRI or CT scan with contrast, which shows a ring-enhancing lesion with surrounding edema (Fig. 21–1). Blood and CSF rarely yield the causative organism. Because of risk of herniation (and low yield of identifying the infectious organism), LP is not indicated. For definitive diagnosis, surgical drainage with cultures is required.

Antibiotic therapy should be tailored to the specific culture and sensitivity results. If the cultures are negative (which can occur in 20% of patients), empiric antibiotic therapy should be aimed at broad coverage

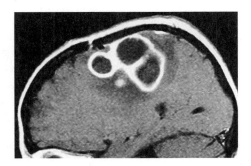

Figure 21–1 Parasagittal MRI showing a multilocular brain abscess. The MRI was performed with gadolinium and shows ring enhancement of the lesion with surrounding edema. (Reproduced with permission from Ginsberg L. Lecture notes on neurology. Malden, MA: Blackwell Science, 1999:121.)

because most abscesses contain multiple organisms. The usual empiric antibiotic regimen includes metronidazole (for anaerobic coverage) and either penicillin or a third-generation cephalosporin (for coverage of streptococci and anaerobes). Surgical drainage of the abscess facilitates treatment, although antibiotics must be continued for 6 to 8 weeks.

◆ KEY POINTS ◆

1. Brain abscess appears as a ring-enhancing lesion on MRI or CT scan.

NEUROSYPHILIS

Syphilis is caused by the spirochete *Treponema pallidum* and is spread either sexually or vertically from mother to child. There are three stages of syphilis. Primary syphilis is characterized by painless chancres that can last 2 to 8 weeks after exposure. Typically, they appear within 3 weeks of infection. Secondary syphilis occurs 2 to 12 weeks after contact and can present with fever, malaise, and generalized lymphadenopathy. Neurologic complications occur in 1% to 2% of patients and most often consist of meningitis or cranial neuropathies, especially loss of hearing. This stage is followed by a latent period of months to many years.

In 30% of untreated patients, tertiary syphilis will develop. Manifestations include chronic syphilitic meningitis that can be associated with brain infarcts due to associated arteritis. General paresis, another neurologic manifestation of tertiary syphilis, is caused by invasion of the brain by the spirochetes and results in Argyll Robertson pupils (small irregular pupils that accommodate but do not react to light) and an encephalitis or dementia. Another manifestation of neurosyphilis is tabes dorsalis, characterized by a sensory ataxia with lightning pains (see Chapter 22). Patients typically have absent knee and ankle reflexes, a positive Romberg sign, and impairment of proprioception because of impairment of dorsal column function. There can also be associated urinary or fecal incontinence. Charcot joints are caused by trophic changes from pain and temperature loss.

Diagnosis is commonly made using treponemal and nontreponemal serologic tests. The fluorescent treponemal antibody (FTA) test is the most commonly used treponemal test. Nontreponemal tests include the rapid plasma reagin (RPR) and Venereal Disease Research Laboratory (VDRL) tests, which detect antibodies to membrane lipids of the treponemal spirochete. Because the nontreponemal tests are very sensitive but not very specific (i.e., they have a high false-positive rate), they are typically used as screening tests. If they are positive, the FTA can be performed to confirm infection. A negative FTA test virtually excludes neurosyphilis. If the test is positive in a patient with signs and symptoms of neurosyphilis, CSF analysis must be done to look for lymphocytic pleocytosis, increased protein, or a reactive CSF-VDRL test.

Treatment should be started in patients with a positive serum FTA and any of the above CSF abnormalities. High-dose intravenous penicillin G is the drug of choice.

◆ KEY POINTS ◆

1. Neurologic manifestations of syphilis can occur in secondary or tertiary syphilis.
2. Tabes dorsalis occurs in tertiary syphilis.

LYME DISEASE

Lyme disease is caused by the spirochete *Borrelia burgdorferi* and is transmitted by the deer tick. Lyme disease is the leading tick-borne disease in Europe and the United States. Clinical symptoms are varied and can involve multiple systems, including dermatologic, cardiac, rheumatologic, and neurologic systems. Neurologic manifestations include lymphocytic meningitis, cranial neuropathy (most commonly a unilateral or bilateral seventh nerve palsy), and painful inflammation of nerve roots.

Diagnosis is supported by erythema chronicum migrans, which is a gradually progressive circular rash with central clearing. The rash typically appears within 3 to 4 weeks of exposure in 60% to 80% of patients and can last days to weeks. Because of the small size of the deer tick species *Ixodes*, patients are often unaware of the tick exposure. Therefore, a history of exposure can be helpful in making the diagnosis but is not necessary. Because some patients do not have all the above signs

or symptoms, diagnosis often depends on serologic testing for antibody against *B. burgdorferi*. In order to prove infection of the nervous system, CSF (in addition to serum) must be obtained for antibody testing. A CSF to serum antibody ratio greater than 1 indicates active CNS infection. Additionally, CSF may show a lymphocytic pleocytosis and mild elevation of protein.

For patients with severe symptoms, treatment is with intravenous antibiotics such as ceftriaxone. If symptoms are mild (i.e., facial weakness) oral antibiotics such as amoxicillin or doxycycline can be used.

◆ KEY POINTS ◆

1. Lyme disease is caused by the spirochete *Borrelia burgdorferi*.

VIRAL INFECTIONS

Meningitis or encephalitis are the typical acute presentations of viral infections of the CNS. Viral meningitis is caused by the inflammatory response of leptomeningeal cells to viral infection. The clinical presentation can be identical to that of bacterial meningitis, with fever, headache, neck stiffness, nausea, and photophobia. If the infection involves the brain parenchyma itself, this is called *encephalitis*; when the meninges and brain are both involved, the term *meningoencephalitis* is used. Because the brain parenchyma itself is affected in encephalitis, the patient can have an altered level of consciousness, cognitive or behavioral abnormalities, focal neurologic deficits, or seizures.

The most common causes of epidemic viral meningitis and encephalitis are the enteroviruses, such as coxsackievirus and echovirus, and the arboviruses, such as eastern equine encephalitis, western equine encephalitis, Venezuelan equine encephalitis, St. Louis encephalitis, and California encephalitis. Meningitis caused by enteroviruses and arboviruses is more common in the summer. Less common causes are herpes simplex virus (HSV), cytomegalovirus, Epstein-Barr virus, and varicella-zoster virus.

Diagnosis of viral meningitis is aided by imaging studies such as MRI that can help exclude alternative diagnoses (such as a mass lesion) for the alteration in alertness, cognition, and behavior. In HSV infection,

TABLE 21–2

Cerebrospinal Fluid Profiles of Meningitis

Etiology	Cell Type	Protein	Glucose
Bacterial	Polymorphonuclear leukocytes	Elevated	Decreased
Tuberculosis	Lymphocytes	Elevated	Decreased
Viral	Lymphocytes or monocytes	Elevated	Normal
Fungal	Lymphocytes	Elevated	Very decreased

the MRI often shows contrast enhancement and edema of the temporal lobes. Electroencephalogram can also be helpful and may show sharp wave discharges in the temporal lobes in the case of HSV infection. LP should be performed for CSF analysis, which provides the best laboratory clue for a viral infection of the CNS or meninges (Table 21–2). In contrast to that of bacterial meningitis, the CSF profile for viral meningitis shows a lymphocytic or monocytic pleocytosis, especially after 48 hours (neutrophils can be present initially), elevated protein, and a normal glucose level. The Gram stain will be negative, so viral meningitis is sometimes referred to as *aseptic meningitis*. It is often difficult to determine a specific viral etiology. Serologic and CSF viral cultures can aid the diagnosis, and newer techniques such as polymerase chain reaction (PCR), which is available for several viruses, can often be helpful. Unfortunately, a definitive etiology is often not found.

Treatment for viral meningitis is mainly supportive, since there are no specific treatments for most viral infections. However, if HSV infection is suspected, the treatment should begin promptly with IV acyclovir even while tests are pending because mortality is close to 70% in untreated cases.

Viral infections of the nervous system can also affect other sites, such as the spinal cord (myelitis), nerves (neuritis), nerve roots (radiculitis), and muscle (myositis). For example, herpes zoster (shingles) is a common manifestation of reactivated varicella-zoster virus in the dorsal root ganglion. A sensation of burning pain is usually followed by eruption of a vesicular rash in a dermatomal pattern that most commonly involves the trunk or the face, particularly the first division of the fifth cranial nerve. Treatment is typically supportive, with analgesics for pain. Oral acyclovir should be used when the infection involves the cornea or involves the

ear with hearing impairment and facial paralysis (Ramsay Hunt syndrome). Patients with herpes zoster who are immunocompromised should be treated with IV acyclovir. The role of corticosteroids is unclear at this time, but they may reduce pain early in the course of the illness.

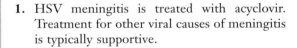

◆   **KEY POINTS**   ◆

1. HSV meningitis is treated with acyclovir. Treatment for other viral causes of meningitis is typically supportive.

PROGRESSIVE MULTIFOCAL LEUKOENCEPHALOPATHY

Progressive multifocal leukoencephalopathy is a demyelinating disease caused by the JC virus. It is a rare disease but occurs more commonly in immunocompromised individuals such as those with Hodgkin's disease, other lymphomas, leukemia, or acquired immunodeficiency syndrome (AIDS). Typically, there are multifocal areas of demyelination, more prominent in the subcortical white matter of the brain.

Clinically, onset of symptoms is subacute or chronic and can include focal signs such as hemiplegia or visual field abnormalities. Dementia can be present in the later stages. Definitive diagnosis is made by brain biopsy, but MRI can show non-enhancing patchy white matter abnormalities. CSF examination is usually normal. Currently, there is no specific treatment other than supportive management, and most patients die within 1 year.

FUNGAL INFECTIONS

Fungal infections of the CNS tend to arise in immuno-compromised patients. They have become more common recently because of the AIDS epidemic and newer immunosuppressive medical treatments. Fungi are eukaryotic organisms that reproduce by budding (yeasts) or by forming hyphae (molds). The most common fungi that cause CNS infections are *Cryptococcus neoformans* and *Coccidioides immitis*. Less common fungal infections of the CNS are *Histoplasma capsulatum* and *Candida* species, among others.

Cryptococcus is the most common cause of fungal meningitis. Cryptococcosis can present with chronic headache, increased intracranial pressure, or cranial nerve signs. Infection occurs by inhalation of *Cryptococcus*, present in soil and pigeon excrement. CSF analysis demonstrates a lymphocytic pleocytosis, very low glucose, and an elevated protein level. The organism can be identified in the CSF with an India ink preparation, but false negatives can occur. In this case, latex agglutination for the cryptococcal antigen can be tested for in the CSF; this test is highly sensitive and specific. Definitive diagnosis is made by a positive CSF culture. Treatment is with amphotericin B and flucytosine.

Coccidioides immitis is the second most common cause of fungal meningitis. Coccidioidomycosis is also caused by inhalation. Infections are more common in the southwestern United States and Mexico. Diagnosis is by CSF culture, with a CSF profile similar to that for cryptococcosis. Treatment is with intravenous and intrathecal amphotericin B.

TOXOPLASMOSIS

Toxoplasmosis is caused by the intracellular parasite *Toxoplasma gondii*. Cats are the definitive host for the parasite, but it can infect a variety of animals, including humans. Humans can be exposed to the parasite either through ingesting soil contaminated with cat feces or by consuming undercooked meat of infected animals. Once ingested, the cysts have a propensity to affect the CNS. Toxoplasmosis can also occur congenitally as one of the TORCH (toxoplasmosis, other agents, rubella, cytomegalovirus, herpes simplex) infections that can be acquired in utero from the first trimester until delivery. In the adult population with AIDS, toxoplasmosis is the most common cause for an intracranial mass lesion. Therefore, the clinical presentation is one of focal neurologic signs accompanied by fever, headache, and mental status changes.

CT or MRI with contrast reveals a ring-enhancing lesion with mass effect, and multiple lesions are usually present. The lesions are typically located in the basal ganglia or at the gray–white matter junction. Antibodies to *T. gondii* help support the diagnosis by proving prior exposure to the parasite. In AIDS patients, diagnosis is often presumptive after an imaging study is obtained. Treatment with pyrimethamine, sulfadiazine, and folinic acid should be continued for 4 to 6 weeks, followed by life-long maintenance therapy with the same medications to help prevent recurrence. If there is no clinical and radiologic improvement after 2 weeks, alternative diagnoses such as primary CNS lymphoma (see Chapter 19) should be considered. Brain biopsy may need to be performed in order to obtain a tissue diagnosis.

CYSTICERCOSIS

Cysticercosis is caused by the pork tapeworm *Taenia solium* when it forms cysts in tissues. Brain involvement is common and occurs in 50% to 70% of all cases. Cysticercosis is the most common parasitic infection of the CNS and is particularly common in Mexico, Central and South America, and Asia.

The most common presentations of cysticercosis are seizures, increased intracranial pressure with headaches, or meningitis. CT or MRI helps make the diagnosis and can show ring-enhancing cystic lesions or small parenchymal calcifications representing calcified cysts. CSF examination may be normal but can show pleocytosis (usually mononuclear), increased protein, and low glucose in cases where meningeal signs are present.

Treatment involves symptomatic management using anticonvulsants to control seizures and shunting to control hydrocephalus if present. Albendazole is used to kill the parasite, and oral steroids are sometimes used to suppress the ensuing inflammatory reaction and edema.

◆ KEY POINTS ◆

1. Cysticercosis is the most common parasitic infection of the CNS. It is particularly common in Mexico, Central and South America, and Asia.

22

Disorders of the Spinal Cord

Because the clinical presentations are diverse, spinal cord disorders can be challenging to the clinician. The diversity in presentation is due, in part, to the functional anatomy of the spinal cord, where sensory and motor systems are in proximity to one another. In order to understand the clinical manifestations of spinal cord disorders, one must understand the anatomy of the spinal cord.

ANATOMY

The spinal cord is the caudal continuation of the lower brainstem. It begins at the foramen magnum and ends at the filum terminale. Below the T12 level, the spinal cord tapers rapidly, forming the conus medullaris that signifies the end of the spinal cord at approximately the L1 level. The lumbar and sacral nerve roots must project downward before they can exit laterally at their appropriate levels. This collection of nerve roots is the cauda equina (horse's tail).

The vascular supply to the spinal cord consists of a single anterior spinal artery and two posterior spinal arteries. The vertebral arteries each extend one branch downward and fuse to form the anterior spinal artery. The anterior spinal artery supplies blood to the anterior two-thirds of the spinal cord. The posterior spinal arteries, which also arise from the vertebral arteries, supply blood to the posterior one-third of the spinal cord, that is, the dorsal columns.

The spinal cord is divided grossly into gray and white matter. The gray matter contains the dorsal (posterior) and ventral (anterior) horns. The dorsal horn contains the cell bodies of neurons involved in the sensory system, and the ventral horn contains the cell bodies for the motor system. The intermediolateral cell column is located in between the dorsal and ventral horns, extends from C8 to L1, and contains the preganglionic cell bodies for the sympathetic nervous system. The white matter in the spinal cord is composed of the myelinated axons of the motor and sensory systems.

Motor Pathways

In the spinal cord, the corticospinal tract begins at the junction of the medulla and the top of the spinal cord, just below the decussation of the medullary pyramids (Fig. 22–1). Two main motor pathways are used for voluntary movement: the lateral corticospinal tract and the ventral corticospinal tract. The lateral corticospinal tract is the major motor pathway and is organized in a somatotopic fashion, with the fibers that innervate the motor neurons to the leg located laterally. Approximately 20% of the corticospinal fibers do not cross in the medulla. These fibers travel in the ventral corticospinal tract, cross in the spinal cord in the white matter anterior to the central canal, and then synapse on motor neurons in the ventral horn.

Clinical signs of corticospinal tract dysfunction include upper motor neuron signs such as enhanced

CORTICOSPINAL TRACT

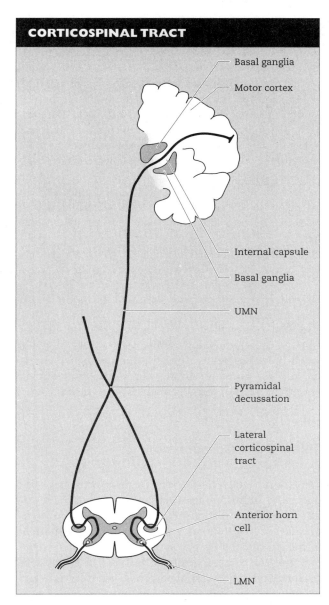

Figure 22–1 Diagram of the corticospinal tract from the cortex to the ventral horn. UMN, upper motor neuron; LMN, lower motor neuron. (Reproduced with permission from Ginsberg L. Lecture notes on neurology, 7th ed. Malden, MA: Blackwell Science, 1999:41.)

reflexes, increased tone, presence of extensor plantar response (Babinski sign), and weakness.

Other motor pathways exist, such as the rubrospinal and vestibulospinal tracts. However, they are not as significant clinically as the corticospinal tract for localizing lesions in the spinal cord.

Sensory Pathways

The major sensory pathways in the spinal cord are the spinothalamic tract and the dorsal columns (Fig. 22–2). Pain and temperature sensations are relayed to the brain by the spinothalamic tracts. First, painful stimuli are relayed to the spinal cord by small, thinly myelinated and unmyelinated fibers. The nerve fibers typically ascend two or three segments before synapsing in the dorsal horn. The fibers then cross to the other side of the cord in the anterior commissure and ascend in the lateral spinothalamic tract to the thalamus. Therefore, a lesion of the spinothalamic tract results in a loss of temperature and pain sensation on the opposite side of the body below the lesion. The spinothalamic tract is somatotopically organized, with the fibers innervating the sacrum and legs located laterally and the fibers innervating the arms located medially.

The dorsal columns relay information concerning joint position sense (proprioception) and two-point dis-

SPINAL CORD (TRANSVERSE)

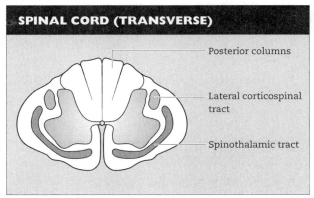

Figure 22–2 Transverse section of the spinal cord showing the sensory pathways. The posterior columns relay information concerning proprioception and two-point discrimination. The spinothalamic tracts relay pain and temperature information. (Reproduced with permission from Ginsberg L. Lecture notes on neurology, 7th ed. Malden, MA: Blackwell Science, 1999:129.)

crimination. Light touch is relayed not only by the dorsal columns but also by the ventral spinothalamic tracts. Likewise, vibratory sense is probably relayed by several pathways in addition to the dorsal columns.

The dorsal columns are composed of two fiber tracts on each side of the spinal cord; the fasciculus gracilis relays information from the legs, whereas the fasciculus cuneatus relays information from the arms. These fiber tracts are organized somatotopically, with the leg fibers located medially because the incoming fibers from the arms push the fibers from the legs toward the middle of the cord.

The fibers in the dorsal columns do not synapse and cross the midline until they reach the gracile or cuneate nuclei in the medulla. Thus, a lesion of the spinal cord affecting the dorsal columns results in loss of joint position sense and fine two-point discrimination on the same side of the body as the lesion. Also, patients sometimes complain of tingling paresthesias or a bandlike sensation in the extremities below the lesion.

◆ KEY POINTS ◆

1. The dorsal horn contains neurons involved in the sensory system.

2. The ventral horn contains the cell bodies of the motor neurons.

3. Corticospinal tract dysfunction results in enhanced reflexes, increased tone, Babinski sign, and weakness.

4. The spinothalamic tract relays pain and temperature.

5. Dorsal columns relay joint position sense and two-point discrimination.

SPINAL CORD SYNDROMES

Armed with knowledge of the anatomy of the spinal cord, one can localize lesions to the spinal cord and compare patterns of findings with known spinal cord syndromes in order to gain clues to the pathophysiology of the spinal lesion.

Complete Spinal Cord Transection

Complete transection of the spinal cord interrupts the sensory and motor pathways on both sides of the spinal cord. Causes of complete transection include trauma, cord compression from a large tumor or hematoma, and transverse myelitis. In the acute phase immediately following spinal transection, there is a period of "spinal shock" that can last days to weeks. During this period, reflexes and tone can be decreased or absent. At the resolution of spinal shock, the reflexes will become hyperexcitable, and tone will increase to the point of spasticity as expected. Because the entire cord is transected, there is complete loss of pain and temperature sense, joint position sense, and voluntary motor strength in all parts of the body below the lesion. For example, a lesion involving the C2 cord level results in quadriplegia with sensory loss over the whole body and occiput of the head. Facial sensation is preserved because the trigeminal system (fifth cranial nerve) is intact. Spinal transection below T1 will allow for complete use of the arms. Lesions of the lumbar and sacral cord result in varying degrees of paraplegia and sensory loss in the lower extremities.

Spinal transection at any level results in bladder and bowel dysfunction with concomitant loss of rectal sphincter tone. Initially, during spinal shock, the bladder becomes atonic, which results in urinary retention. If the sacral spinal cord is intact, reflex emptying of the bladder occurs several weeks after the transection.

Spinal Cord Compression

Cord compression from a mass such as a tumor, hematoma, epidural abscess, or herniated disc can present with the findings discussed above, but the severity of symptoms varies depending on the degree of compression. Cervical spondylosis, a degenerative condition of the spinal column, is common in older patients and may present with some of the features of spinal cord compression. On examination, one can typically find varying degrees of weakness in all four extremities in an upper motor neuron pattern as well as impairment of spinothalamic and dorsal column function.

Brown-Séquard Syndrome

Brown-Séquard syndrome results from a unilateral lesion or hemisection of the spinal cord. Because only one-half of the spinal cord is lesioned, weakness is present only on the side of the body ipsilateral to the lesion. Additionally, there is loss of ipsilateral joint position sense and contralateral pain and temperature below the lesion. The most common cause of Brown-Séquard syndrome is trauma, but spinal metastases causing cord compression can be responsible infrequently.

Central Cord Syndrome

Lesions within the spinal cord itself (intramedullary) cause a central cord syndrome. The most common causes are tumors, syringomyelia, and hematomyelia. Syringomyelia is a fluid-filled cavity in the spinal cord (Fig. 22–3), whereas hematomyelia is a region of hemorrhage in the spinal cord. These lesions can occur anywhere in the spinal cord, but syringomyelia and hematomyelia occur more commonly in the cervical region.

The typical scenario for central cord syndrome occurs when the anterior commissure, which contains the crossing fibers of the spinothalamic tract, is disrupted. If the lesion is in the cervical cord, this results in loss of pain and temperature in a capelike distribution because the crossing fibers from both arms are affected (Fig. 22–4). Dorsal column function is usually spared.

If the intramedullary lesion is large enough and extends into the ventral horn, segmental weakness can result because of involvement of the anterior horn cells. Additionally, if the lesion were to grow even larger, it could affect the spinothalamic tracts on both sides of the spinal cord. Because of the somatotopic organization of the spinothalamic tracts, with fibers from the sacrum located laterally, there can be sacral sparing since only the medial portions of the spinothalamic tract are compressed from the outwardly growing lesion. In lesions of this size, the corticospinal tracts are often involved bilaterally, resulting in weakness and spasticity below the lesion.

Anterior Spinal Artery Syndrome

Because the single anterior spinal artery supplies blood to the anterior two-thirds of the spinal cord, compromise of this artery can cause infarction of the ventral

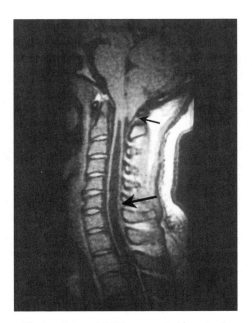

Figure 22–3 Sagittal MRI scan of the spinal cord showing a hypointense region in the middle of the cord that represents a fluid-filled syrinx cavity (large black arrow). (Reproduced with permission from Ginsberg L. Lecture notes on neurology, 7th ed. Malden, MA: Blackwell Science, 1999:131.)

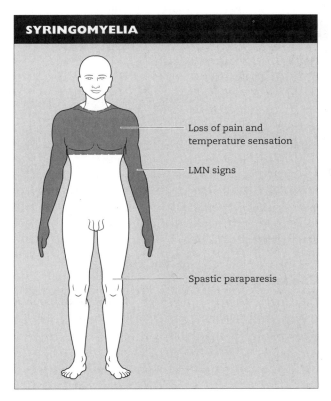

SYRINGOMYELIA

Loss of pain and temperature sensation

LMN signs

Spastic paraparesis

Figure 22–4 Clinical features of syringomyelia. (Reproduced with permission from Ginsberg L. Lecture notes on neurology, 7th ed. Malden, MA: Blackwell Science, 1999:132.)

(anterior) horns and the spinothalamic tracts. Therefore, corticospinal and spinothalamic dysfunction occurs below the site of infarction. Since the posterior spinal arteries supply the dorsal columns, joint position sense and two-point discrimination are unaffected.

Anterior Horn Cell Syndromes

The most important of the anterior horn cell disorders is amyotrophic lateral sclerosis (ALS), which has both upper and lower motor neuron signs because of involvement of the corticospinal tracts and motor neurons, respectively (see Chapter 23 for more detail). Pure anterior horn cell degeneration occurs in spinal muscular atrophy such as Werdnig-Hoffman disease, an inheritable disorder that typically presents in infancy. Kugelberg-Welander disease is another type of spinal muscular atrophy that can be either inherited or sporadic. It typically presents in early childhood or adolescence.

Poliomyelitis is a historically important cause for weakness because the virus has a predilection for affecting the anterior horn cells. Because of vaccination, this infection is now rare in developed countries.

Diseases of the Posterior and Lateral Columns

Vitamin B_{12} deficiency results in combined dysfunction of the dorsal columns and corticospinal tracts, also referred to as subacute combined degeneration. This results in a spastic ataxic gait. The spasticity is caused by corticospinal dysfunction, and the sensory ataxia by loss of proprioception from the dorsal column involvement.

Isolated dorsal column dysfunction can result from tabes dorsalis, a late complication of syphilis. The dorsal columns can degenerate to the point where the patient develops a sensory ataxia.

Lesions of the Conus Medullaris and Cauda Equina

Pathologic lesions in the area of the cauda equina and conus medullaris cause similar symptoms due to involvement of multiple lumbar and sacral nerve roots. Typically, the patient has radicular pain, loss of sensation in the buttocks and legs, and leg weakness. Lesions of the conus medullaris typically also have more prominent symptoms of bowel, bladder, and sexual dysfunction.

◆ KEY POINTS ◆

1. Spinal cord transection results in bilateral weakness and complete sensory loss below the lesion.

2. "Spinal shock" is the acute phase of spinal cord transection, and tone can be flaccid with decreased reflexes.

3. Brown-Séquard syndrome is a hemisection of the cord with ipsilateral weakness and loss of proprioception and contralateral loss of pain and temperature.

4. Syringomyelia of the cervical spinal cord resulting in a capelike distribution of pain and temperature loss is the classic example of central cord syndrome.

5. Anterior spinal artery infarction results in bilateral weakness and loss of pain perception with sparing of dorsal column function.

6. ALS and polio are examples of motor neuron diseases that affect the anterior horn cell.

7. Vitamin B_{12} deficiency results in subacute combined degeneration (involvement of dorsal columns and corticospinal tracts).

8. Tabes dorsalis is caused by late syphilis infection and results in impairment of dorsal column function.

23

The Peripheral Nervous System

The peripheral nervous system consists of cranial nerves, spinal roots, peripheral nerves, muscles, and autonomic ganglia. The system consists of afferent fibers that connect the sensory receptors to the central nervous system, and efferent fibers that connect the central nervous system to the effector apparatus.

Three classically described pathologic changes affect peripheral nerve axons (Fig. 23–1):

- *Wallerian degeneration:* After axon and myelin injury, a distal disintegration of axon and myelin occurs.
- *Neuronal (or axonal) degeneration:* Develops after damage to the cell body of the neuron, resulting in the distal dying of the axon and subsequent loss of myelin.
- *Demyelination:* A loss of the myelin sheath.

APPROACH TO PERIPHERAL NEUROPATHY

The goals in the evaluation of peripheral neuropathy (PN) are to localize the site of pathology to the axon, myelin sheath, cell body, or vascular structures (Table 23–1); identify the cause; and prescribe treatment when available.

Start by determining the types of symptoms (motor, sensory, autonomic, or mixed); the distribution of weakness (proximal or distal, symmetric or asymmetric); the nature and distribution of sensory involvement (small fiber, large fiber, or mixed); and the evolution of the condition (acute, subacute, or chronic).

The next step is to recognize a pattern of peripheral neuropathy that will help to determine the etiology of the disease (Table 23–2). Finally, characterize the primary pathologic process by using electrodiagnostic studies, including nerve conduction studies and electromyography (EMG).

◆ KEY POINTS ◆

1. The symptoms associated with involvement of small nerve fibers are neuropathic pain (described as aching, shooting, throbbing, or burning); temperature sensations; and autonomic dysfunction (cardiac arrhythmias, orthostatic hypotension, impotence, and constipation).

2. The symptoms associated with involvement of large fibers are loss of vibration and joint position sense, weakness, denervation with fasciculations, and loss of deep tendon reflexes.

INVESTIGATION OF THE PERIPHERAL NERVOUS SYSTEM

Additional investigation requires a logical and rational approach. Order tests sequentially, guided by the

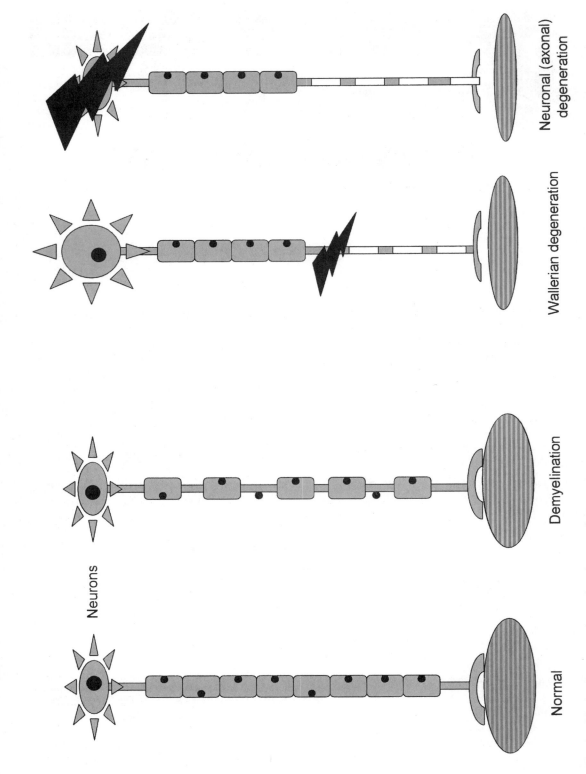

Figure 23–1   Patterns of peripheral nerve damage.

TABLE 23–1

Approach to the Classification of Peripheral Neuropathy

Functional involvement
  Motor
  Sensory
    Small fiber
    Large fiber
    Small and large fiber
  Autonomic

Anatomic distribution
  Asymmetric
  Symmetric
  Upper extremity
  Lower extremity

Temporal course
  Acute: GBS, porphyria, diphtheria, polio, toxins
    (thallium, lead, arsenic, Adriamycin), paraneoplastic,
    uremia, vasculitis
  Subacute: deficiency states (vitamins B_1 and B_{12}),
    toxins, uremia, diabetes, sarcoidosis,
    paraneoplastic, vasculitis, drugs
  Chronic: CIDP, diabetes, uremia
  Relapsing: CIDP

Pathologic mechanism
  Axonal
  Demyelination
  Combined neuropathy

GBS, Guillain-Barré syndrome; CIDP, chronic inflammatory demyelinating polyneuropathy.

clinical and electrodiagnostic study findings. In general, first-line tests include complete blood cell count (CBC), erythrocyte sedimentation rate (ESR), and rheumatoid profiles (for collagen disease, leukemia, vasculitis); renal function and liver function tests (uremic and hepatic neuropathy); glucose and Hb-A1C levels (diabetes); vitamin B_{12} and folate levels (neuropathy with macrocytosis); thyroid function tests (hypothyroid neuropathy); serum protein electrophoresis and urine protein electrophoresis (dysproteinemias, monoclonal gammopathy, lymphoma, amyloidosis).

Second-line tests include urine porphobilinogen (acute intermittent porphyria); urine heavy metals such as lead, arsenic, and mercury; arsenic in hair and nails (arsenic neuropathy); hepatitis-B Ag, antineutrophil cytoplasmic antibodies (Wegener's granulomatosis); computed tomography (CT) scan of chest (cancer survey carcinomatous neuropathy); cerebrospinal fluid (CSF) protein (Guillain-Barré syndrome, chronic inflammatory demyelinating polyneuropathy); CSF pleocytosis (Lyme disease, AIDS, paraneoplastic); serum HIV (AIDS neuropathy); Lyme titers; anti-Hu Ab (paraneoplastic); anti-GM1, MAG Ab (autoimmune neuropathy); and genetic testing for hereditary neuropathy.

Electrodiagnostic studies include nerve conduction studies and EMG. A nerve biopsy should be performed when indicated.

◆ KEY POINTS ◆

1. A mnemonic for the most common causes of peripheral neuropathies is DANG THE RAPIST: Diabetes, Alcohol, Nutritional, Guillain-Barré, Trauma, Hereditary, Environmental (toxins and drugs), Rheumatic (vascular), Amyloid, Paraneoplastic, Infections, Systemic disease, and Tumors.

2. *Polyneuropathy* refers to symmetric involvement of the peripheral nerves, usually involving legs more than arms and distal more than proximal segments, the "stocking-glove" pattern.

3. *Mononeuropathy* refers to involvement of a single nerve, for example, median neuropathy at the wrist, also known as carpal tunnel syndrome.

4. *Mononeuropathy multiplex* refers to involvement of individual nerves in a multifocal distribution.

5. *Radiculopathy* refers to involvement of nerve roots (Table 23–3).

EPIDEMIOLOGY

The prevalence of PN among patients with no recognized exposure to diseases or neurotoxic agents is 2%. Diabetes mellitus is the most common risk factor, followed by alcoholism, nonalcoholic liver disease,

TABLE 23–2

Pattern-Recognition Approach to Peripheral Neuropathy

Pattern	Possible Causes
Symmetric proximal and distal weakness with sensory loss	GBS, CIDP
Symmetric distal weakness with sensory loss	Drug-induced, toxic, and metabolic neuropathies; hereditary neuropathies; amyloidosis
Asymmetric distal weakness with sensory loss	
Multiple nerves	Vasculitis; HNPP; infections such as leprosy, Lyme disease, sarcoidosis, and HIV
Single nerve	Compressive mononeuropathy and radiculopathy
Asymmetric distal weakness without sensory loss	Motor neuron disease, multifocal motor neuropathy
Asymmetric proximal and distal weakness with sensory loss	Polyradiculopathy or plexopathy, meningeal carcinomatosis or lymphomatosis, HNPP, hereditary neuropathies
Symmetric sensory loss without weakness	Cryptogenic sensory polyneuropathy; metabolic, drug-induced, or toxic neuropathies; leprosy
Asymmetric proprioceptive sensory loss without weakness	Sensory neuronopathies (ganglionopathies); consider paraneoplastic, Sjögren's syndrome, vitamin B_6 toxicity, HIV-related sensory neuronopathies, cis-platinum toxicity
Autonomic symptoms and signs	Diabetes mellitus, amyloidosis, GBS, vincristine, porphyria, HIV-related autonomic neuropathy, idiopathic pandysautonomia

GBS, Guillain-Barré syndrome; CIDP, chronic inflammatory demyelinating polyneuropathy; HNPP, hereditary neuropathy with liability to pressure palsy; HIV, human immunodeficiency virus.

and malignancy. Among patients with one or two risk factors, the prevalence is 12% and 17%, respectively.

The most common causes of PN in the United States are hereditary (30%), followed by cryptogenic (23%), diabetes mellitus (15%), multifocal motor neuropathy (MMN), vitamin B_{12} deficiency, and drugs (Table 23–4).

IMMUNE-MEDIATED NEUROPATHIES

Guillain-Barré Syndrome (Acute Inflammatory Demyelinating Polyneuropathy)

Epidemiology
There are 1 to 2 cases of Guillain-Barré syndrome (GBS) per 100,000 population per year. Males and

females are at equal risk. Adults are more frequently affected than children. Of those affected, 5% will die of the illness, but more than 85% make an excellent recovery.

Pathogenesis
In 75% of patients, neurologic symptoms are preceded by an acute infection (usually respiratory or gastrointestinal). Twenty-five percent of cases in the United States are preceded by infection with *Campylobacter jejuni*, and another 25% by a herpesvirus infection, most frequently cytomegalovirus or Epstein-Barr virus. Acute inflammatory demyelinating polyneuropathy (AIDP) is considered an autoimmune disease, with neural targets represented by gangliosides. Many antiganglioside antibodies (Abs) are found in GBS, with the most

TABLE 23–3

Root Syndromes

Segment	Sensation	Motor Deficit	Reflexes
Cervical			
C5	Pain in lateral shoulder; sensory loss over deltoid	Paresis of deltoid, supraspinatus, and biceps	Impairment of biceps reflex
C6	Radial side of the arm to thumb	Paresis of biceps and brachioradialis	Impairment or loss of biceps reflex
C7	Between 2nd and 4th finger	Triceps, wrist extensors and flexors, pectoralis major muscles	Impairment or loss of triceps reflex
Lumbosacral			
L3	Often none; lateral area if any	Quadriceps and anterior tibial paresis; adductor may be affected (differentiates from femoral neuropathy)	Loss of knee jerk; loss or impaired adductor reflex
L4	Medial leg below knee to medial malleolus	Quadriceps and anterior tibial muscles; inversion of the foot	Decreased knee jerk
L5	Dorsum of foot to great toe	Extensor hallucis longus and extensor digitorum longus	None
S1	Lateral border of the foot	Plantar flexion and eversion of foot	Decreased or absent ankle jerk

frequent being anti-GM1, but anti-GD1a, anti-GQ1b, anti-GD1b, and others are found as well.

Clinical Features

GBS presents as a rapidly evolving, ascending areflexic motor paralysis with or without sensory disturbances. Initial symptoms often consist of tingling and pins-and-needle sensations in the feet, sometimes with lower back pain. Weakness evolves over hours to days, reaching its worst within 30 days (usually by 14 days). Bulbar weakness and respiratory muscle paralysis may occur. Tendon reflexes usually disappear after 3 days. Over 50% of patients develop facial weakness, and 10% have extraocular muscle paralysis. Pain is common. Autonomic dysfunction may be present, with orthostatic hypotension, transient hypertension, and cardiac arrhythmias.

The Miller-Fisher variant is characterized by gait ataxia, areflexia, and external ophthalmoplegia, usually without limb weakness. Nerve conduction studies are normal, and anti-GQ1b Abs are positive in 90% of cases.

Diagnosis

Albumino-cytologic dissociation in the CSF (elevated protein but few or no cells) is characteristic. Usually the CSF protein rises after the first 3 days. Early electro-diagnostic findings may include prolonged distal latencies, variably prolonged or absent F waves, and possible conduction block. Early EMG changes include decreased motor unit recruitment. Routine laboratory evaluation should include CBC, ESR, liver function tests, and HIV test. The differential diagnosis includes spinal cord disease such as transverse myelitis, and acute neuromuscular junction problems or myopathy.

Treatment

Patients should be hospitalized. Monitoring should include frequent measurement of the forced vital capacity (FVC) and negative inspiratory pressure. An FVC

TABLE 23–4

Classification of Peripheral Neuropathy by Etiology

Immune-mediated neuropathies
  Guillain-Barré syndrome
  CIDP
  Multifocal motor neuropathy
  Neuropathy associated with monoclonal neuropathy
  Immune-mediated ataxic neuropathies, including carcinomatous sensory neuropathy, sensory ganglionitis
    associated with Sjögren's syndrome, and idiopathic sensory ganglionitis
  Vasculitic neuropathies: Rheumatoid arthritis, Sjögren's syndrome, hepatitis B, Lyme disease, HIV, etc.

Metabolic neuropathies
  Diabetic neuropathy
  Thyroid disease
  Hepatic neuropathy
  Uremic neuropathy
  Porphyric neuropathy (acute intermittent porphyria)
  Vitamin deficiency (B_1, B_6, B_{12})
  Critical care neuropathy
Hereditary neuropathies
  Charcot-Marie-Tooth disease
  Amyloid neuropathies
  Hereditary neuropathy with liability to pressure palsy
  Hereditary sensory and autonomic neuropathies
  Neuropathy with leukodystrophy (metachromatic leukodystrophy, Krabbe's disease, adrenoleukoneuropathy)

Toxic neuropathies
  Metals: Arsenic, lead, mercury, thallium
  Drugs: vincristine, cisplatin, antiretrovirals
  Substance abuse: alcohol, glue inhalation, nitrous oxide inhalation
  Industrial poisons: acrylamide, carbon disulfide, cyanide, ethylene, hexacarbon, organophosphorous,
    trichloroethylene (trigeminal neuropathy)

Neuropathies associated with infections
  HIV
  Lyme neuropathy
  Leprosy (the most frequent infectious cause of neuropathy in the world)
  CMV and herpes

Entrapment and compressive neuropathies
  Upper extremity: carpal tunnel syndrome or median neuropathy, ulnar neuropathy, radial neuropathy
  Lower extremity: femoral and peroneal neuropathies, among others

CIDP, chronic inflammatory demyelinating polyneuropathy; HIV, human immunodeficiency virus; CMV, cytomegalovirus.

below 15 mL/kg warrants transfer to the intensive care unit and likely intubation. Medical treatment includes intravenous immunoglobulin (IVIg) or plasmapheresis (equally effective). IV steroids are not proven to be beneficial.

◆ KEY POINTS ◆

1. GBS is characterized by ascending paralysis and absent deep tendon reflexes.
2. CSF shows albumino-cytologic dissociation: few cells and high protein.
3. Measurement of FVC is important to decide whether the patient needs to be intubated (<15 mL/kg of body weight).
4. Treatment includes IVIg or plasmapheresis.

Chronic Inflammatory Demyelinating Polyneuropathy

Chronic inflammatory demyelinating polyneuropathy (CIDP) is sometimes called chronic GBS. Although there are many similarities, the two conditions differ in time course and in the absence of identifiable antecedent events for CIDP.

Epidemiology
CIDP may occur at any age, typically in adults between 40 and 60 years of age.

Clinical Features
Patients experience a slowly evolving, usually painless weakness beginning in the legs, with widespread areflexia and loss of vibratory sense (larger fiber). Weakness of neck flexors is often present.

Diagnosis
Diagnosis of CIDP is supported by clinical features, time course, relapses, prominent demyelinating features in nerve conduction studies, and CSF protein elevation.

Management
Unlike GBS, CIDP responds to steroids alone. Some patients respond to plasmapheresis and others to intravenous immunoglobulin. Treatment is required for many years.

◆ KEY POINTS ◆

1. CIDP is a chronic, relapsing, inflammatory polyneuropathy.
2. Weakness and areflexia are characteristic symptoms.
3. Treatment is with steroids. IVIg has also shown to be effective.

Multifocal Motor Neuropathy

MMN is an uncommon disorder characterized by a pure motor multiple mononeuropathy. It usually occurs in young adults. There is a slight male predominance. Evidence supports an immune-mediated mechanism.

Clinical Features
Patients present with a slowly progressive, asymmetric, predominantly distal limb weakness that begins in the arms. Weakness develops in the distribution of individual nerves rather than following a spinal myotome, and weakness can be severe in muscles with relatively normal bulk. Reflexes are spared in less affected muscles. Minor sensory symptoms are common. Objective sensory deficits, upper motor neuron findings, and cranial nerve findings are usually absent.

Diagnosis
Diagnosis is made by clinical features plus electrodiagnostic studies demonstrating partial conduction block in motor nerves in areas not prone to compression. CSF protein is usually normal. Nerve biopsy is nonspecific. A very high IgM anti-GM1 is found in 60% to 80% of patients with MMN. It is important to recognize and distinguish MMN from typical motor neuron disease because MMN responds to IVIg or immunosuppressive drug therapy such as cyclophosphamide.

◆ KEY POINTS ◆

1. MMN is characterized by a pure motor multiple mononeuropathy.
2. Positive anti-GM1 antibodies are present in 60% to 80% of patients.
3. MMN responds to IVIg and immunosuppressive therapy.

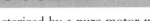

Neuropathies Associated with Myeloma and Other Monoclonal Gammopathies

Approximately 10% of peripheral neuropathies are associated with serum monoclonal gammopathy (M-protein) that reacts with myelin-associated glycoprotein (MAG). One-third of those patients have multiple myeloma, amyloidosis, macroglobulinemia, cryoglobulinemia, lymphoma, or leukemia.

Clinical Features
The neuropathy develops as a symmetric sensory (early) and motor (late) neuropathy that usually affects the legs more than the arms. This neuropathy has prominent large-fiber sensory loss and sensory ataxia, as well as weakness.

Diagnosis
Electrodiagnostic studies show demyelination.

Treatment
Treatment depends on the cause. If the neuropathy is due to a plasmacytoma, excision and radiation of the tumor can be curative. In other cases, plasmapheresis may have some benefit.

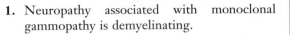

◆ KEY POINTS ◆

1. Neuropathy associated with monoclonal gammopathy is demyelinating.

METABOLIC NEUROPATHIES

Diabetic Polyneuropathy

Diabetic polyneuropathy is the most common and important diabetic neuropathy (Table 23–5) and is a common complication of diabetes mellitus.

Epidemiology
The prevalence of diabetic neuropathy increases with the duration of diabetes (usually developing after 5 to 10 years of the disease), but it is uncommon at the time of diagnosis of diabetes mellitus. The pathogenesis is not clear, but hyperglycemia is required.

Clinical Features
Patients may report neuropathic pain and dysesthesias. More characteristic is a distal, symmetric, slowly

---

TABLE 23–5

Diabetic Neuropathies

Type	Comments
Chronic progressive distal symmetric diabetic polyneuropathy	Mixed sensory-autonomic-motor polyneuropathy; variants include small-fiber (painful, usually spontaneous burning pain), large-fiber (ataxic), and autonomic
Diabetic proximal motor neuropathy (diabetic amyotrophy)	Severe thigh and back pain, followed within weeks by mild to severe hip and thigh muscle weakness with muscle atrophy; usually affects older type 2 diabetic patients
Acute axonal diabetic polyneuropathy (intensely painful acute or subacute progressive symmetric sensory axonal peripheral neuropathy)	Diabetic neuropathic cachexia (with worsening hyperglycemia); insulin neuritis (with improved hyperglycemia)
Diabetic mononeuropathy, radiculopathy, and polyradiculopathy	Can present with cranial neuropathy (third, fourth, and sixth nerves), multisegmental truncal radiculopathy, or limb mononeuropathy
Focal compression neuropathies associated with diabetes	Diabetic patients are more susceptible to compression neuropathies, such as median nerve at the wrist, ulnar nerve at the elbow, and peroneal nerve at the knee

progressive sensory loss in the lower extremities (stocking distribution, beginning with toes and feet before hands). There is some autonomic insufficiency. Weakness is a late feature.

Diagnosis

Diagnosis is straightforward in established diabetes with typical clinical findings. It is an axonal polyneuropathy, usually involving small and large fibers.

Treatment

Glucose control is the best treatment. Symptomatic management of neuropathic pain includes the use of nonsteroidal anti-inflammatory drugs (NSAIDs), tricyclic antidepressants, or anticonvulsants such as gabapentin or carbamazepine.

◆ KEY POINTS ◆

1. Diabetic polyneuropathy is the most common and important of the diabetic neuropathies.
2. It usually involves small and large fibers.
3. The neuropathy is distal symmetric with stocking-glove distribution.
4. Neuropathic pain responds to anticonvulsants such as gabapentin or carbamazepine.

Other Metabolic Neuropathies

Uremic Neuropathy

Uremic neuropathy is a symmetric, distally predominant, motor-sensory axonal polyneuropathy. Foot drop and leg weakness are major manifestations.

Porphyric Neuropathy

Porphyric neuropathy is usually associated with acute intermittent porphyria. It is an acute or subacute motor-sensory axonal PN manifested by paresthesias and dysesthesias of the extremities with rapidly evolving weakness or paralysis (mimicking the axonal form of GBS), with areflexia and abdominal pain.

Critical Care Neuropathies

Critical care neuropathies develop in 50% of patients with severe medical illness who have been in the intensive care unit for more than 2 weeks. The etiology is unclear. Electrodiagnostic studies show an axonal neuropathy.

HEREDITARY NEUROPATHIES

Hereditary neuropathies are the most prevalent inherited neurologic disease and also the most common cause of polyneuropathy in patients referred to a neurologic clinic.

Charcot-Marie-Tooth disease (CMT) is the most common inherited PN, with an estimated prevalence of 40 per 100,000 adults and 19 per 100,000 children. CMT typically presents in adolescence with symmetric, slowly progressive distal muscular atrophy of the legs and feet, and in most cases, eventually involves the hands. The age of onset, severity, and rate of progression can vary, even within the same family.

◆ KEY POINTS ◆

1. CMT-2 is the only axonal motor neuropathy of the CMT family; the others are primarily demyelinating.
2. Hereditary sensory and autonomic neuropathy (HSAN) is a hereditary neuropathy that affects autonomic sensory or motor nerves.
3. There is no specific drug or gene therapy for hereditary neuropathies.

INFECTIOUS NEUROPATHIES

PN occurs in a number of infections, including viral, bacterial, parasitic, and prion disease. These peripheral neuropathies are beyond the scope of this chapter.

HIV Neuropathies

HIV neuropathies include the following:

- *Distal sensory polyneuropathy:* Occurs in more than 30% of patients with AIDS. It may be HIV related, nucleoside treatment related, or due to neurotoxic medications.

- *Mononeuropathy and multiple mononeuropathies:* Usually occur late in the illness, sometimes associated with superimposed infection (herpes, cytomegalovirus, hepatitis C, and syphilis), lymphomatous infiltration, or necrotizing vasculitis.

TABLE 23-6

Entrapment Neuropathies

Nerve	Clinical Features	Examination	Etiology
Upper extremities			
Median nerve (at the wrist is called carpal tunnel syndrome)	Numbness or tingling involving one or more of the first four digits. Occasionally the entire hand is involved. May awake from sleep with symptoms. Usually exacerbated by exercise. Occasionally pain in the whole forearm.	Weakness and atrophy of the thenar muscle, particularly the APB. Decreased sensation in the volar aspect of the first four digits. Tinel's and Phalen's signs may be present.	Compression of the median nerve at the wrist within the space known as the carpal tunnel. Flexor tenosynovitis; vascular lesions; ganglion cysts; tumoral calcinosis; pseudoarthrosis; and systemic illness, including hypothyroidism, acromegaly, and SLE.
Ulnar nerve (at the elbow)	Paresthesias and pain in the fifth digit and the medial half of the fourth. May also involve the median forearm and elbow. Difficulty spreading the fingers.	Weakness relevant in the FDI and ADM. Atrophy may be present in those muscles, and claw hand deformity may develop.	Compression of the ulnar nerve at the elbow. Remote elbow trauma predisposes to later development of entrapment neuropathy in the elbow region. Arthritis can also produce it.
Radial nerve	Weakness of radial-innervated muscles and sensory loss on the dorsal aspects of the hand.	Weakness includes triceps, brachioradialis, supinator, and the wrist and finger extensors. The triceps is affected by axillary compression, but spared by spiral groove compression. Weakness of wrist extensors causes wrist drop.	Compression of the radial nerve at the level of the axilla, the spiral groove, and the forearm (posterior interosseous neuropathy). At the axilla level can be secondary to use of crutches. At the spiral groove is likely to occur when an individual falls asleep with an arm hanging over a chair (Saturday night palsy).

Lower extremities

Meralgia paresthetica (lateral cutaneous nerve of the thigh)	Burning sensation and variable loss of sensation over the anterolateral part of the thigh.	Area of sensory change over the lateral aspect of the thigh. Palpation of the inguinal ligament can usually detect an area of tenderness and precipitate symptoms. No motor involvement.	Caused by entrapment of the lateral cutaneous nerve near the inguinal ligament (but can be caused by compression in the retroperitoneal space, trauma to the thigh, etc.).
Femoral neuropathy	Leg weakness on attempting to stand or walk. Pain in the anterior thigh is common.	Exam reveals weakness of the quadriceps muscles; absent or diminished patellar reflex; and sensory loss over the anterior thigh and, with saphenous nerve involvement, the medial leg/foot. Adductors intact (differentiates from an L2-3 radiculopathy).	Usually trauma from surgery, stretch injury (prolonged lithotomy position in childbirth). Diabetes mellitus and other inflammatory processes.
Peroneal neuropathy	Patient usually presents with foot drop with minimal sensory complaints.	Weakness of extensor hallucis longus, tibialis anterior (foot dorsiflexion), and the peroneal muscles (eversion of the foot). Sensory loss over the dorsal part of the foot is mild.	Entrapment of the peroneal nerve between the neck of the fibula and the insertion of the peroneus longus muscle. Usually due to trauma and compression.

APB, abductor pollicis brevis; SLE, systemic lupus erythematosus; FDI, first dorsal interosseous; ADM, abductor digiti minimi.

- *Acute inflammatory demyelinating polyneuropathy:* Similar to GBS and responsive to plasmapheresis and IVIg.
- *Lumbosacral polyradiculoneuropathy:* Uncommon, but usually associated with cytomegalovirus infection. It is a devastating complication and presents as a rapidly progressive flaccid paraparesis, with sphincter dysfunction, perineal sensory loss, and lower limb areflexia.

Neuropathy of Leprosy

Leprosy is one of the most common neuropathies in the world. It is caused by *Mycobacterium leprae.* Sensory neuropathy is more common than motor. It usually presents as a mononeuropathy multiplex or mononeuropathies with predilection for the ulnar and peroneal nerve. In general, it respects the muscle stretch reflexes. It is usually associated with hypertrophy of the peripheral nerve. Axonal damage, myelin changes, and nerve fiber loss are cardinal features in lepromatous leprosy.

ENTRAPMENT NEUROPATHIES

Entrapment neuropathies are a common group of mononeuropathies produced by nerve entrapment (pressure, stretch, friction, and so forth). They are reviewed in Table 23–6.

◆ KEY POINTS ◆

1. Leprosy is one of the most common neuropathies in the world.
2. HIV neuropathies are common.
3. Tips to remember about peripheral neuropathies are found in Table 23–7.

MOTOR NEURON DISEASES

Several different diseases are characterized by progressive degeneration and loss of motor neurons in

---

TABLE 23–7

Tips to Remember about Peripheral Neuropathies

Neuropathies that may begin proximally
   Sensory: porphyria, occasionally CMT and Tangier disease
   Motor: GBS, CIDP, diabetes

Neuropathies that may begin in the arms rather than legs: lead toxicity, leprosy, sarcoidosis, porphyria, entrapment, diabetes, vasculitic neuropathy, Tangier disease

Predominantly sensory neuropathies
   Autoimmune: Miller-Fisher syndrome, IgM paraproteinemia, paraneoplastic, Sjögren's syndrome
   Toxic: pyridoxine and doxorubicin
   Infectious: diphtheria, HIV
   Nutritional: vitamin E deficiency

Neuropathies that are predominantly motor: GBS, porphyria, and multifocal motor neuropathy

Neuropathy associated with cranial nerve involvement: diphtheria, sarcoid, diabetes, GBS, Sjögren's syndrome, polyarteritis nodosa, Lyme disease, porphyria, Refsum's disease, syphilis, arsenic

Causes of mononeuritis multiplex: trauma, diabetes, vasculitis, leprosy, HIV, Lyme disease, sarcoidosis, tumor infiltration, lymphoid granulomatosis, HNPP

Neuropathies associated with palpable peripheral nerves: CMT and Dejerine-Sottas, amyloidosis, Refsum's disease, leprosy, acromegaly, neurofibromatosis

---

CMT, Charcot-Marie-Tooth disease; GBS, Guillain-Barré syndrome; CIDP, chronic inflammatory demyelinating polyneuropathy; HIV, human immunodeficiency virus; HNPP, hereditary sensory neuropathy with liability to pressure palsy.

the spinal cord. They are considered motor neuron diseases.

Amyotrophic Lateral Sclerosis (Lou Gehrig's Disease)

Amyotrophic lateral sclerosis (ALS) has its onset in middle and late life. Five percent of cases are familial in an autosomal dominant pattern (20% map to chromosome 21).

Clinically, there are lower and upper motor neuron findings (LMN and UMN, respectively). Weakness, wasting and fasciculations are LMN signs of MND; hyperreflexia, Babinski sign, clonus, and spasticity are UMN signs. These findings may coexist in the same limbs. Weakness may commence in the legs, hands, proximal arms, or oropharynx (with dysarthria or dysphagia).

Diagnosis is primarily clinical. The course is relentless and progressive, without remissions. Death results usually in the first 5 years. Electrodiagnostic studies show active denervation in at least three limbs.

The major treatment is supportive. Riluzole is a glutamate inhibitor that prolongs life by 3 to 6 months but does not improve function or quality of life.

◆ KEY POINTS ◆

1. ALS is characterized by the presence of UMN and LMN symptoms in the same limbs.
2. Death usually occurs within 5 years.
3. EMG shows clear evidence of denervation.
4. Riluzole is the only proven treatment to prolong life marginally.

24

Disorders of the Neuromuscular Junction and Skeletal Muscle

Myasthenia gravis (MG) and the Lambert-Eaton myasthenic syndrome (LEMS) are the two most common diseases of the neuromuscular junction (NMJ) (Table 24–1). Fatigable muscle weakness is the defining clinical feature of these disorders and is most important in distinguishing these NMJ disorders from the myopathies. There is no single defining clinical feature of disorders of skeletal muscle. However, the selective involvement of particular groups of muscles (i.e., focal patterned weakness) is highly suggestive of a myopathic process.

Nerve and muscle have both undergone structural and functional specialization at their point of contact, the NMJ. At the presynaptic bouton, secretory vesicles containing acetylcholine (ACh) are concentrated at active zones formed by clusters of P/Q-type voltage-gated calcium channels. Across the synaptic cleft, the muscle membrane is thrown into folds at what is known as the *muscle end plate*. Acetylcholine receptors are clustered at the peaks of these folds. Depolarization of the nerve terminal, mediated by a Na^+-dependent action potential, leads to activation of the voltage-gated calcium channels, which in turns leads to calcium influx into the presynaptic bouton. The rise in intracellular calcium triggers the release of ACh via a process known as *exocytosis*, whereby the synaptic vesicles dock at the active zones and then fuse with the presynaptic membrane to release their contents into the synaptic cleft.

The ACh molecules diffuse across the cleft to bind to the acetylcholine receptors. This generates an inward Na^+ current through the acetylcholine receptor ion pore that leads to depolarization of the muscle end plate. This in turn triggers activation of voltage-dependent sodium channels that line the troughs of the end-plate membrane folds, resulting in muscle contraction. The action of ACh is terminated by its metabolism via acetylcholinesterase in the synaptic cleft.

MYASTHENIA GRAVIS

Acquired MG is an immunologic disorder in which antibodies are directed against the postsynaptic (muscle) nicotinic acetylcholine receptor (nAChR). Blockade and down-regulation of these nAChRs reduces the probability that a nerve impulse will generate a muscle action potential.

Epidemiology

MG is the most common disorder of NMJ transmission. Younger-onset MG is often associated with thymic hyperplasia, whereas thymoma is more commonly seen in later-onset disease.

Pathophysiology

In acquired MG, antibodies are directed against the postsynaptic nAChR. These antibodies directly block

TABLE 24–1

Disorders of the Neuromuscular Junction and Skeletal Muscle

Disease	Clinical Phenotype	Dysfunctional Protein
Myasthenia gravis	Fatigable proximal muscle weakness; prominent ocular and bulbar involvement	Nicotinic acetylcholine receptor
Lambert-Eaton myasthenic syndrome	Fatigable proximal muscle weakness; ocular and bulbar involvement rare; prominent autonomic symptoms	P/Q-type voltage-gated calcium channel
Duchenne and Becker muscular dystrophy	Childhood onset of proximal muscle weakness, including neck flexors; no ocular or bulbar involvement	Dystrophin
Limb-girdle muscular dystrophy	Proximal muscle weakness; no ocular or bulbar involvement	Sarcoglycan
Myotonic dystrophy	Distal muscle weakness and stiffness; myotonia; systemic features (ptosis, balding, etc.)	Dystrophica myotonia protein kinase (DMPK)
Emery-Dreifuss muscular dystrophy	Early onset of joint contractures; humeroperoneal pattern of muscle weakness	Emerin and lamin A/C
Hypokalemic periodic paralysis	Episodes of generalized weakness lasting hours to days	Skeletal muscle L-type voltage-gated calcium channel
Hyperkalemic periodic paralysis	Episodes of generalized weakness lasting minutes to hours	Voltage-gated sodium channel

the binding of ACh and lead to a complement-mediated attack and internalization of receptors. The end result is distortion of the end plate with loss of the normal postjunctional folds and a reduction in the concentration of the receptors. Thus, even though ACh is released normally from the presynaptic bouton, its effect at the end plate is reduced, with the result that the nerve impulse is less likely to generate a muscle action potential. This failure of neuromuscular transmission is what accounts for the weakness in patients with MG. Fatigability occurs because of depletion of presynaptic vesicles with sustained activity.

Clinical Features

Fatigable muscle weakness is characteristic. The specific symptoms depend on the distribution of this weakness. Ocular involvement is most common, manifesting as ptosis and diplopia. The pupils are never involved. Bulbar muscle weakness is next most frequent and man-

ifests as dysarthria or dysphagia. Limb weakness is usually proximal and symmetrical. Symptoms are typically worse with sustained activity or toward the end of the day. Deep tendon reflexes are usually preserved.

Most patients with MG have generalized disease, but as many as 15% may have restricted ocular involvement. The sensitivity of the ancillary diagnostic tests depends on whether the disease is generalized or restricted.

Diagnosis

The diagnosis of MG is primarily clinical, but support for the diagnosis may be obtained from various tests. Edrophonium chloride (Tensilon) is an anti-acetylcholinesterase. It is administered intravenously and the patient observed for improvement in muscle strength. Antibodies against the nAChR may be detected in about 80% of patients with generalized MG and 55% of patients with ocular MG. Elevated titers confirm the diagnosis, but negative titers do not exclude it. Seronegative MG is clinically indistinguishable from seropositive disease. Repetitive nerve stimulation reveals a decremental response that is seen more commonly in proximal muscles. Single-fiber electromyography is the most sensitive clinical test of neuromuscular transmission. The characteristic finding in MG is increased jitter.

Management

Anti-acetylcholinesterase drugs such as pyridostigmine inhibit the synaptic degradation of acetylcholine and thus prolong its effect. Although pyridostigmine provides adequate symptomatic therapy for many patients with MG, it does not affect the underlying immunopathology. Immune-modulating therapy thus serves as the mainstay for most patients with MG. There are few controlled trials of immunosuppressive therapy, but steroids, steroid-sparing agents such as azathioprine and cyclosporin, plasmapheresis, and intravenous immunoglobulin (IVIg) have all been used with some success. Plasmapheresis and IVIg provide rapid (but relatively short-lived) immunosuppression for patients with severe disease. Steroids and steroid-sparing agents are the mainstay for long-term immune therapy. The place and timing of thymectomy are not clear, but most would agree that it will facilitate easier immunosuppression in young patients.

◆ KEY POINTS ◆

1. MG is mediated by antibodies directed against the nAChR.
2. It presents with fatigable muscle weakness.
3. MG is treated with acetylcholinesterase inhibitors and steroids.

LAMBERT-EATON MYASTHENIC SYNDROME

Epidemiology

LEMS is an uncommon condition that is usually associated with an underlying small cell lung carcinoma. It is caused by antibodies directed against the presynaptic P/Q-type voltage-gated calcium channel. By reducing presynaptic calcium entry, these antibodies reduce ACh release, leading to weakness.

Clinical Features

Patients present with fatigable proximal weakness. Deep tendon reflexes are reduced or absent. In contrast to MG, bulbar and ocular symptoms are rare, but autonomic complaints (dry eyes, dry mouth, and impotence) are common. The characteristic finding is that of muscle facilitation. With brief intense exercise, muscle strength increases and reflexes may briefly appear. Fatigue develops with sustained activity.

Diagnosis

The presence of elevated anti-voltage-gated calcium channel antibody titers together with an incremental response on repetitive nerve conduction studies helps to establish the diagnosis.

Management

The diagnosis of LEMS should prompt a thorough search for an underlying malignancy, even though a tumor is not always found. Initial therapy is directed at the underlying malignancy; in many patients, no further therapy is required. Steroids, azathioprine, intravenous immunoglobulin, and plasmapheresis have all been used, but with less success than in MG.

◆ KEY POINTS ◆

1. LEMS is mediated by anti-voltage-gated calcium channel antibodies.
2. It has a strong association with underlying small cell lung cancer.

SKELETAL MUSCLE DISORDERS

Disorders of skeletal muscle are a diverse group of conditions that do not lend themselves to easy classification. Discussion of these diseases is further complicated by the array of terminology commonly used. A few words of clarification may help. *Myopathy* is a nonspecific term used to refer to disorders of skeletal muscle. Muscular *dystrophy* refers to a group of hereditary conditions in which muscle biopsy demonstrates *dystrophic* changes (fiber splitting, increased connective tissues). *Myotonia* is a state of increased muscle contraction or impaired relaxation. The term *congenital* indicates onset of clinical disease in the early infantile period. *Myositis* implies an inflammatory process.

Broadly speaking, it is still useful to think of these disorders as inherited or acquired. The inherited disorders encompass the muscular dystrophies, the congenital myopathies, and the channelopathies as well as the metabolic and mitochondrial myopathies. The acquired disorders include the inflammatory myopathies, endocrine and drug- or toxin-induced myopathies, and a group of myopathies associated with other systemic illnesses. With recent advances in molecular genetics, there has been a shift toward thinking about and classifying at least the hereditary disorders on the basis of the underlying molecular defect. The approach adopted herein is an attempt to synthesize clinical classification with newly acquired knowledge of the genetic basis of many of the inherited skeletal muscle disorders.

DYSTROPHINOPATHIES

Duchenne muscular dystrophy (DMD) and Becker muscular dystrophy (BMD) result from different mutations of the same gene, dystrophin, and are thus said to be *allelic*.

Clinical Features

DMD and BMD should be thought of as a single disorder representing a spectrum of severity, with DMD more severe than BMD. Inheritance is X-linked, and onset is usually in childhood. The child may use an arm to push down on his thighs when arising from the floor (Gower's sign), and there may be pseudohypertrophy of the calf muscles. Proximal muscle weakness, including neck flexors, predominates; there is usually sparing of ocular and bulbar muscles. DMD is relentlessly progressive, with the child becoming wheelchair bound by the age of 10 or 12. Although primarily a disorder of skeletal muscle, cardiac and gastrointestinal smooth muscle involvement, as well as central nervous system involvement, is common. In DMD death usually occurs around age 20 because of respiratory insufficiency and aspiration. Life expectancy is also reduced in BMD.

Diagnosis

The creatine kinase (CK) level is typically markedly elevated in DMD and moderately so in BMD. A normal CK level provides strong presumptive evidence against the diagnosis. Muscle biopsy shows dystrophic features, with absent or reduced staining for dystrophin.

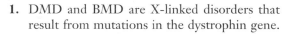

◆ KEY POINTS ◆

1. DMD and BMD are X-linked disorders that result from mutations in the dystrophin gene.
2. They present clinically as proximal muscle weakness in young boys.

LIMB-GIRDLE MUSCULAR DYSTROPHIES

The limb-girdle muscular dystrophies are a group of hereditary conditions in which the proximal muscles of the arms and legs are predominantly affected.

Clinical Features

Most of these disorders are characterized by weakness of the limb-girdle muscles with relative sparing of facial, extraocular, and pharyngeal musculature. Cardiomyopathy is less frequent than in the dystrophinopathies.

Classification

There are both autosomal dominant and recessive varieties. Some are due to mutations in proteins known as the sarcoglycans, which form part of the multimolecular dystrophin-associated glycoprotein complex.

Diagnosis

CK level is usually elevated. The EMG is myopathic, and biopsy demonstrates nonspecific dystrophic changes. Immunohistochemistry with antibodies directed against the various sarcoglycan proteins may help to distinguish the different limb-girdle muscular dystrophies.

◆ KEY POINTS ◆

1. Limb-girdle muscular dystrophies are characterized clinically by shoulder and hip girdle weakness with relative sparing of extraocular, pharyngeal, and facial muscles.
2. They affect both boys and girls and may resemble the dystrophinopathies, requiring muscle biopsy for differentiation.

MYOTONIC DYSTROPHY

The classic form of myotonic dystrophy is the most common inherited skeletal muscle disorder that affects adults. Inheritance is autosomal dominant and the genetic defect is an unstable CTG expansion in the DMPK (dystrophia myotonica protein kinase) gene.

Clinical Features

Myotonic dystrophy is a multisystem disease. Weakness and stiffness of distal muscles are usually the presenting symptoms in young adults. Action and percussion myotonia are often present. Proximal weakness develops later in the course of the disease. Systemic findings include cataracts, ptosis, arrhythmias, dysphagia (from esophageal myotonia), insulin resistance, testicular atrophy, and frontal balding. Neurobehavioral features (changes in affect, personality, and motivation) as well as cognitive dysfunction are also commonly observed.

Diagnosis and Management

CK level is usually normal or only mildly elevated. Electromyography demonstrates myotonia. DNA testing for the CTG expansion is now available. There is no specific treatment for the muscle weakness, but drugs such as phenytoin and carbamazepine may reduce the myotonia. Management is otherwise supportive.

◆ **KEY POINTS** ◆

1. Myotonic dystrophy is the most common adult-onset muscular dystrophy.
2. It is a trinucleotide repeat disorder.
3. Myotonic dystrophy presents with distal muscle weakness and myotonia.

CHANNELOPATHIES

The channelopathies are a group of disorders characterized by ion channel dysfunction. The clinical manifestations are determined by the specific ion channel involved.

The periodic paralyses (PP) are autosomal dominant conditions that derive their designation from their cardinal manifestation, episodic muscle weakness. Attacks of weakness are usually associated with a change in serum potassium concentration, and they are therefore classified accordingly into hypokalemic and hyperkalemic varieties. Hypokalemic PP is the result of a mutation in the pore-forming α_{1S}-subunit of the skeletal muscle calcium channel that secondarily results in dysfunction of the Na^+/K^+ ATPase. Hyperkalemic PP results from mutations in the skeletal muscle voltage-gated sodium channel.

◆ **KEY POINTS** ◆

1. The periodic paralyses are characterized by episodic muscle weakness.
2. They are caused by mutations in skeletal muscle membrane ion channels.

MITOCHONDRIAL MYOPATHIES

The mitochondrial myopathies are a heterogeneous group of disorders with systemic manifestations.

Inheritance

Mitochondrial DNA is entirely maternally inherited; this is, therefore, the usual mode of inheritance for mitochondrial disorders. However, given that over 90% of mitochondrial proteins are encoded by nuclear genes, virtually all other patterns of inheritance may also occur.

Clinical Features

A number of characteristic syndromes have been identified. These include myoclonic epilepsy with ragged red fibers (MERRF); mitochondrial myopathy, encephalopathy, lactic acidosis, and stroke-like episodes (MELAS); progressive external ophthalmoplegia (PEO); and the Kearns-Sayre syndrome.

Diagnosis

There are no characteristic clinical or electrophysiologic findings in the mitochondrial myopathies, but a common finding is the co-occurrence of a myopathy and a peripheral neuropathy. Serum or CSF lactate and pyruvate are often increased. The histopathologic changes are also nonspecific and include the presence of ragged red fibers and variability of cytochrome oxidase staining.

DISTAL MYOPATHIES

The distal myopathies are group of largely hereditary conditions in which muscle weakness at onset is predominantly distal. Distal muscle weakness, however, may occur atypically in acquired disorders such as polymyositis and inclusion body myositis in which weakness is usually more proximal. Distal weakness may also occur in some of the other muscular dystrophies (e.g., fascioscapulohumeral, scapuloperoneal, and Emery-Dreifuss humeroperoneal).

INFLAMMATORY MYOPATHIES

The noninfectious immune-mediated inflammatory myopathies include polymyositis (PM), dermatomyositis (DM), and inclusion body myositis (IBM).

Clinical Features

PM, DM, and IBM are all characterized by proximal (usually symmetrical) muscle weakness. Pharyngeal and neck flexor muscles may be affected, but facial and respiratory muscles are usually spared. IBM is often only diagnosed when patients thought to have PM fail to respond to steroids. However, early selective involvement of forearm and finger flexors, as well as ankle extensors, should arouse suspicion of this diagnosis. Dermatomyositis is distinguishable by the associated purplish discoloration of the eyelids (heliotrope) and papular erythematous scaly lesions over the knuckles (Gottren's patch). Extramuscular manifestations include dysphagia, heart conduction defects, congestive cardiac failure, and interstitial lung disease.

Pathogenesis

DM is a microangiopathic disorder in which antibodies and complement are directed primarily against intramuscular blood vessels. Inflammation is secondary to muscle ischemia. PM and IBM are mediated via antigen-directed cytotoxic T-cell processes.

Diagnosis

CK level is almost invariably elevated. EMG demonstrates myopathic changes (often with accompanying denervation changes secondary to muscle fiber necrosis). The histology of each myopathy is characteristic, with rimmed vacuoles required for the diagnosis of IBM.

Management

Corticosteroids are the mainstay of treatment in PM and DM, but are of no benefit in IBM.

ENDOCRINE AND DRUG- OR TOXIN-INDUCED MYOPATHIES

Thyrotoxic Myopathy

Although weakness is rarely the presenting complaint of patients with thyrotoxicosis, it is found on examination in many patients. Proximal muscle weakness and atrophy are usually the dominant clinical features, but rarely distal weakness may be the earliest manifestation. Bulbar and respiratory muscle involvement is uncommon. Reflexes may be brisk, reflecting shortened relax-

TABLE 24–2

Drug- or Toxin-Induced Myopathies

Disorder	Drug or Toxin	Clinical Syndrome
Necrotizing myopathy	HMG-CoA reductase inhibitors; cyclosporin; propofol; alcohol	Acute or insidious onset of proximal muscle weakness; CK level typically elevated
Steroid myopathy	Fluorinated glucocorticoids	Proximal muscle weakness; CK level usually normal
Mitochondrial myopathy	Zidovudine	Acute or insidious onset of proximal muscle weakness; CK level normal or only mildly increased
Inflammatory myopathy	Cimetidine; procainamide; L-dopa; phenytoin; lamotrigine; D-penicillamine	Acute onset of proximal muscle weakness; CK level typically increased
Critical illness myopathy	Corticosteroids plus neuromuscular blocking agents in patients with sepsis	Acute or subacute onset of generalized weakness; CK level may be normal or elevated

HMG-CoA, hydroxymethylglutaryl coenzyme A; CK, serum creatinine kinase.

ation time. If Graves disease is the cause of thyrotoxicosis, then the differential diagnosis of muscle weakness should include myasthenia gravis. The pathogenesis of thyrotoxic myopathy is unknown, but may reflect enhanced muscle catabolism. CK level is typically normal, and EMG demonstrates myopathic units. Muscle strength will improve with treatment of the underlying thyrotoxic state, but β-blockers may improve strength acutely.

Hypothyroid Myopathy

Myopathic symptoms develop in about one-third of patients with hypothyroidism. The typical presentation is that of proximal muscle weakness, fatigue, myalgias, and cramps. Reflexes may demonstrate delayed relaxation. There may be an associated distal polyneuropathy. CK level is typically elevated (10 to 100 times normal). EMG shows nonspecific myopathic changes. Weakness usually improves following thyroid replacement, but recovery may lag behind a return to the euthyroid state.

Steroid Myopathy

Myopathy may result from increased glucocorticoids from either endogenous production or exogenous

administration. The latter is more common, and although any synthetic glucocorticoid can cause myopathy, it is more common with the fluorinated compounds (e.g., triamcinolone and dexamethasone). Doses in excess of the equivalent of 30 mg prednisone per day are associated with an increased risk of myopathy. The risk is reduced with alternate-day regimens. Typically, weakness begins after chronic administration of steroids, but may occur within a few weeks. Weakness is predominantly proximal, with sparing of the ocular, bulbar, and facial muscles. CK level is usually normal. EMG is usually normal. Muscle biopsy typically demonstrates type II fiber atrophy, but this finding is nonspecific. Treatment requires a reduction in the steroid dose, switching to an alternative-day regimen or to a non-fluorinated compound.

Drug- or Toxin-Induced Myopathy

Many drugs and toxins have been implicated as the cause of a myopathy. Typically, they produce a syndrome characterized by proximal myopathy and increased serum CK level. Some of the more commonly encountered drugs that induce myopathies are listed in Table 24–2.

◆ KEY POINTS ◆

1. Proximal muscle weakness is frequently found in patients with either hypothyroidism or hyperthyroidism.

2. Proximal myopathy may result from excessive circulating steroids, either from increased endogenous production or exogenous administration.

3. CK level is usually normal in the metabolic myopathies, except for hypothyroidism, in which CK level is typically elevated.

25

Pediatric Neurology

Neurologic disorders in children are commonly encountered by pediatricians and general physicians. Many neurologic diseases that affect infants and children also affect adults, such as infection, epilepsy, inflammatory and demyelinating diseases, peripheral neuropathies, and myopathies; but some are characteristic of early ages, including developmental disorders, malformations, and genetically determined conditions. Seizures are one of the most common neurologic problems in childhood (see Chapter 15).

The history is the most important component of the evaluation of a child with a neurologic problem. It shares the same principles as described for the adult history, but also requires a complete review of the pregnancy, labor, and delivery, especially if a perinatal injury or a congenital infection is suspected.

DEVELOPMENT AND MATURATION

One of the most important elements of the neurologic history is a developmental assessment of the child. The Denver Developmental Screening Test is an efficient and reliable method to assess achievement of developmental milestones. It evaluates four components of development, including gross motor skills, fine motor adaptive skills, language, and personal-social interaction. Table 25–1 summarizes developmental milestones by age. This is based on averages and therefore can only be used with an understanding of the variability among children. Table 25–2 gives a brief description of primitive reflexes and their significance.

EMBRYOGENESIS OF THE CENTRAL NERVOUS SYSTEM

Understanding developmental disorders and malformations requires a basic knowledge of how the central nervous system (CNS) is formed. The basic form of the human CNS is complete by about the sixth week of gestation. The next phases, which include cellular proliferation and migration, are most prominent during the second trimester but continue until term. Myelination peaks during the third trimester but continues until adulthood.

The first neural tissue appears at the end of the third week of embryonic development. The neuroectoderm gives rise to the brain, spinal cord, and peripheral nervous system. The CNS develops from the neural tube. The neural canal is open rostrally in the anterior neuropore and closes at about 24 days; the caudal opening or posterior neuropore closes 2 days later. *Dysraphic defects* are congenital malformations associated with defective neurulation (closing at the neuropores). Failure of the anterior neuropore to close causes anencephaly. *Encephaloceles* are herniation of intracranial contents through a defect in the cranium (crania bifidum). They occur more frequently in the occipital region but may occur in the frontal and parietal areas. Problems with

TABLE 25–1

Developmental Milestones

Age	Adaptive/Fine Motor Skills	Gross Motor Skills	Language	Personal/Social
1 month	Grasp reflex; hand fisted	Raises head slightly when prone	Facial response to sounds	Stares at face
2 months	Follows objects with eyes past midline	Lifts head from prone to 45 degrees	Coos	Smiles in response to others
4 months	Hands open; brings objects to mouth	Sits, head steady; rolls to supine	Laughs and squeals; turns toward voice	Smiles spontaneously
6 months	Palmar grasp of objects; starts transfer of objects	Sits independently; stands with hands held	Babbles (consonant sounds); mimics sounds	Reaches for toys; recognizes strangers
9 months	Pincer grasp; claps hands	Pulls to stand	Says "mama," "dada," nonspecifically; comprehends "no"; associates word and action ("bye-bye," "no," etc.)	Finger-feeds self; waves bye-bye
1 year	Helps to turn pages of book; tower of two blocks	Stands independently; walks with one hand held	2–4 words; follows command with gesture	Points to indicate wants
18 months	Turns pages of book; imitates vertical lines	Walks up steps	10–20 words; points to four body parts; obeys simple commands	Feeds self with spoon; uses cup
2 years	Solves single-piece puzzles	Jumps; kicks ball	Combines 2–3 words; uses "I" and "you"; 50–300 words	Removes coat; verbalizes wants
3 years	Copies circle; draws person with three body parts; imitates horizontal lines; towers of six cubes; draws circles	Throws ball overhand; walks up stairs, alternating feet	Gives full name, age, and sex; names two colors	Toilet trained; puts on shirt and knows front from back
4 years	Counts four objects; identifies some numbers and letters; uses scissors	Hops on one foot	Understands prepositions (under, on, behind, in front of); asks "how" and "why"	Dresses with little assistance; shoes on correct feet
5 years	Prints first name; counts 10 objects; draws triangle; draws person with several parts	Skips, alternating feet	Asks meaning of words; understands conjunctions and past tenses; knows colors	Ties shoes

TABLE 25–2

Special Reflexes

Reflex	Significance	Appears	Disappears
Moro	Elicited by head extension. Two phases: extension and abduction of arms and leg extension, followed by slower abductions of arms. Asymmetry indicates central nervous system disease such as hemiparesis, spinal cord lesion or brachial plexus injury.	Term newborns	3 months
Tonic neck	Turning head, arm and leg extended in the side toward the turn and flexion in the other side (fencing posture). If infant is unable to move out of posture, implies possible brain pathology.	1 month	5 months
Traction response	Lift baby by traction in both hands. Head lag after 6 months is pathologic and indicates hypotonia.	Birth	6 months
Parachute	Elicited by plunging suspended infant downward. Arms should thrust forward symmetrically as if breaking the fall. Also elicited with baby in sitting position and pushed forward. Arms should try to break the fall. Asymmetry suggests hemiparesis, spinal cord lesion, or brachial plexus pathology	6 months	Persists throughout life

closure of the posterior neuropore cause a range of malformations known as *myeloschisis* (myelomeningocele, meningocele, and spina bifida occulta and aperta). During the first gestational month, external agents such as drugs and infections can interfere with the process of neurulation. For example, valproic acid can interfere with closure of both anterior and posterior neuropores, and colchicine can interfere with posterior neuropore closing.

After the fourth week, the primary brain vesicles start to form: prosencephalon, or forebrain; mesencephalon, or midbrain; and rhombencephalon, or hindbrain. This is also the time of formation of midline structures. Interference with normal development during this period may produce agenesis of the corpus callosum, cleft palate, cleft lip, hypertelorism, cycloplegia, and double uvula. Limbs are being developed at the same time; therefore, appendicular abnormalities can occur simultaneously with developmental problems of midline structures.

During the fifth week, the secondary brain vesicles appear. The rhombencephalon divides into myelen-cephalon and metencephalon. The mesencephalon remains undivided, and the forebrain is divided into the diencephalon and the telencephalon. During the second month of gestation the main structures of the forebrain develop. At this same time, facial structures are forming, so abnormalities of forebrain development are often associated with facial defects.

Failure of the prosencephalon to undergo cleavage produces *holoprosencephaly*, in which there is a large single ventricle, the thalamus is poorly developed, and many structures (corpus callosum, falx cerebri, and olfactory structures) are lacking. Patients with holoprosencephaly typically have developmental delay, seizures, and midline facial abnormalities.

The next process in the shaping of the cerebral cortex is the formation of gyri and migration. During peak periods of cellular migration, the hemispheric fissures appear and mold the telencephalic surface into gyri and sulci. The secondary sulci are completed by 32 weeks, and the tertiary sulci are completed during the last month of gestation.

Abnormal patterns of gyri and sulci are caused by disorders of migration. If the gyri fail to form, the cerebral cortex will have a smooth surface, a condition called *lissencephaly*. Unusually large gyri constitute *pachygyria*, and unusually small gyri constitute *microgyria*. Any of these conditions may affect the whole cerebrum or may be localized and even coexist in the same patient. *Schizencephaly* refers to unilateral or bilateral clefts in the cerebral hemispheres due to abnormal morphogenesis.

Porencephaly is the presence of cysts or cavities within the brain that result from development defects or acquired lesions, including infarction.

◆ KEY POINTS ◆

1. The neuroectoderm gives rise to the brain, spinal cord, and peripheral nervous system.
2. The first brain tissue develops in the third week of gestation.
3. Neurulation, vesicle formation, cellular proliferation, migration, and myelination are the different stages necessary for brain formation and function.

CEREBRAL PALSY

Cerebral palsy (CP) refers to a group of static disorders characterized by chronic motor deficit of cerebral origin acquired prenatally, perinatally, or up to 2 years of age.

Cerebral palsy occurs in about 2.7 per 1,000 births. Risk factors for CP include hypoxic-ischemic insult to the brain in the perinatal period, prematurity, low birth weight, chorioamnionitis, prenatal viral infections, and prenatal strokes.

Classification

According to etiology, CP can be congenital, acquired, or genetic. According to the type of motor abnormalities, CP is classified as spastic or hypertonic, flaccid or hypotonic, associated with rigidity or tremor, dyskinetic (athetoid), ataxic, and mixed. The most common form of CP is spastic or hypertonic.

The most commonly used classification is based on the distribution of the affected limbs:

- *Hemiplegic:* Unilateral cerebral damage with spasticity in arm and leg on the contralateral side.
- *Diplegic:* Spasticity in both legs, with relative sparing of arms, even though they are usually involved.
- *Quadriplegic:* Bilateral cerebral damage with involvement of all limbs.

Clinical Features

In general, the clinical manifestations are noted at the latest age of normal walking, about 2 years. In the first week of life, there may be flaccid weakness or asymmetric involvement of the limbs. The infant may have seizures or other abnormalities. In older children, spasticity in the involved limbs, dystonia, and drooling are common presentations.

Diagnosis

The diagnosis of CP is based on the clinical symptoms and signs. The cause may not be determined, but the presence of a static disorder is suggestive. One must rule out other entities that may present with dystonia, ataxia, or spasticity that progress with time (e.g., metabolic disorders, metachromatic leukodystrophy, and movement disorders such as levodopa-responsive dystonia). Magnetic resonance imaging (MRI) is indicated only to exclude other structural causes such as tumor, stroke, or arteriovenous malformations.

Management

In general, a multidisciplinary approach is necessary, with early infant stimulation, physical and occupational therapy, orthopedic and psychological evaluation, and speech therapy. Management will depend on the severity of CP.

◆ KEY POINTS ◆

1. CP is a static disease: It does not progress.
2. It occurs in almost 3 per 1,000 births.
3. The most common abnormality is spasticity.

MENTAL RETARDATION

Another common neurologic condition is mental retardation, defined as below-average general intellectual function with associated deficits in adaptive skill areas (communication, self-care, home living, social skills, self-direction, health and safety, functional academics, leisure, and work) that occurs before age 18. The degree of impairment from mental retardation has a wide range, from profoundly impaired (5%) to mild or borderline retardation (80% to 90%). Mental retardation can be classified according to intelligence quotient (IQ) as mild (IQ = 55 − 70), moderate (IQ = 40 − 55), severe (IQ = 25 − 40) and profound (IQ < 25). The prevalence of mental retardation in industrialized counties is 1% to 3%.

Etiologies

There are many different causes of mental retardation. Among them are prenatal and postnatal trauma (e.g.,

intracerebral hemorrhage and hypoxic-anoxic encephalopathy); congenital and postnatal infection (e.g., congenital rubella, syphilis, cytomegalovirus, toxoplasmosis, and HIV infection); chromosomal abnormalities (e.g., Down syndrome, fragile X syndrome, Angelman's syndrome, Prader-Willi syndrome); chromosomal translocations (e.g., cri du chat syndrome); inherited metabolic disorders (e.g., hypothyroidism, galactosemia, Tay-Sachs disease); and toxic, nutritional, and environmental causes. Table 25–3 summarizes some chromosomal abnormalities associated with mental retardation.

Diagnosis

The diagnosis of mental retardation requires below-average scoring in tests used to assess development and

TABLE 25–3

Mental Retardation Syndromes

Condition	Epidemiology	Genetic Defect	Clinical Characteristics
Fragile X syndrome	Most common inherited form of MR; affects males more than females	Defect in the X chromosome; mutation in the 5′ end of the gene with amplification of a CGG repeat (200 or more copies)	20% of males are normal; 30% of carrier females are mildly affected; moderate mental retardation; behavioral problems; somatic abnormalities: long face, enlarged ears, and macro-orchidism
Prader-Willi syndrome	Uncommon inherited disorder	Absence of segment 11–13 on the long arm of the paternally derived chromosome 15	Mental retardation; decreased muscle tone; short stature; emotional lability and insatiable appetite (obesity)
Angelman's syndrome	Uncommon neurogenetic disorder	Deletion of segment 11–13 on the maternally derived chromosome 15	Mental retardation; abnormal gait; speech impairment; seizures; inappropriate happy behavior that includes laughing, smiling, and excitability (happy puppet syndrome)
Rett's syndrome	Progressive neurodevelopmental disorder; generally affects only females; most common cause of MR in women; incidence of 1 in 10,000 births	Causal gene is MeCP2, found in the long arm of chromosome X (X 28)	Normal development until 6–18 months; a first sign is hypotonia; autistic-like behavior; stereotyped hand movements (wringing and waving); lag in brain and head growth; gait abnormalities; seizures

MR, Mental retardation.

intelligence (e.g., Wechsler Preschool and Primary Scale of Intelligence–Revised, Wechsler Adult Intelligence Scale, and Stanford-Binet, among others); an IQ two standard deviations below the mean (usually < 70, with mean of 100); an adaptive behavior score that is below average (e.g., Vineland Adaptive Behavior Scales); and an abnormal Denver Developmental Screening Test.

It is important to distinguish between mental retardation and developmental delay. The former implies a child with cognitive and adaptive behaviors below average functioning; the latter refers to a child who is not achieving certain developmental skills as quickly as expected.

Treatment

Treatment includes special education and training, starting early in infancy.

◆ **KEY POINTS** ◆

1. Mental retardation implies a below-average cognitive ability and adaptive behavior.

2. Developmental delay implies inability to achieve developmental milestones at the usual age. It is not synonymous with mental retardation.

AUTISTIC SPECTRUM DISORDERS

Autism is conceptualized as a developmental disorder of brain function. Usually, the etiology is unknown. It has a wide range of behavioral consequences referred to as *pervasive developmental disorder*.

Clinical Features

Three major elements identify autistic disorders. Abnormal language is characterized as echolalic, repetitive, and stereotyped. Marked deficiencies in social and communication skills manifest as a lack of attachment to other members of the family and poor social contacts. The last characteristic is a restricted range of behaviors, interests, and activities, with repetitive and stereotyped behaviors such as toe walking, rocking, flapping, banging, and licking.

Diagnosis

The diagnosis is clinical. Differential diagnosis considers other causes of language problems, such as deafness, mental retardation, and seizures (Landau-Kleffner syndrome). *Asperger's disorder* is a variant of autistic disorder that is characterized by social isolation and eccentric behavior during childhood, with normal intelligence and language development.

Treatment

The treatment of autism includes support and behavioral modification.

DEVELOPMENTAL REGRESSION

Developmental regression is defined as a loss of previously attained developmental milestones. It is often related to a progressive disease of the CNS. It is one of the most distressing complaints confronted by pediatricians and neurologists. An extensive battery of diagnostic tests is the wrong approach. A complete history, physical and neurologic examination, and additional tests based on those findings are fundamental in reaching an accurate diagnosis.

Always differentiate regression from developmental delay (see above). Table 25–4 shows common causes of progressive encephalopathy at different ages that can produce developmental delay or regression.

◆ **KEY POINTS** ◆

1. Autistic children have problems with language, social skills, and behavior.

2. Developmental regression represents a major problem in child neurology. A rational approach is needed to reach the diagnosis.

NEUROCUTANEOUS DISORDERS

Neurocutaneous disorders include neurofibromatosis (NF), tuberous sclerosis complex (TSC), Sturge-Weber syndrome, familial telangiectasia, Von Hippel-Lindau disease (hemangioblastoma of the cerebellum), incontinentia pigmenti, and ataxia-telangiectasia.

TABLE 25–4

Causes of Progressive Encephalopathy

Onset before Age 2	Onset after Age 2
Mitochondrial disorders	AIDS
Hypothyroidism	Congenital syphilis
Neurocutaneous syndrome	Subacute sclerosing panencephalitis
Tuberous sclerosis complex	Enzymatic lysosomal disorders
Neurofibromatosis	Gaucher's disease
Gray matter disorders	Gangliosidosis
Infantile ceroid lipofuscinosis	Late-onset Krabbe's disease
Rett's syndrome	Metachromatic leukodystrophy
White matter disorders	Other gray matter disorders
Alexander's disease	Ceroid lipofuscinosis
Canavan's disease	Huntington's disease
Neonatal adrenoleukodystrophy	Mitochondrial disorders (MERRF)
Pelizaeus-Merzbacher disease (peroxisomal disorders)	Other white matter disorders
Disorders of amino acid metabolism	Adrenoleukodystrophy
Homocystinuria	Alexander's disease
Maple syrup urine disease	
Phenylketonuria	
Enzymatic disorders	
Gangliosidosis	
Gaucher's disease	
Krabbe's disease	
Mucopolysaccharidoses	
Metachromatic leukodystrophy	

AIDS, acquired immunodeficiency syndrome; MERRF, myoclonic epilepsy with ragged red fibers.

Tuberous Sclerosis Complex

The incidence of TSC is 1 in 10,000. It is inherited in an autosomal dominant manner, with chromosome 9 being implicated for TSC-1, and chromosome 16 for TSC-2. Hamartin is the gene product for TSC-1, and tuberin the gene product for TSC-2. Both are considered tumor suppressor genes.

The cardinal clinical features are skin lesions (adenoma sebaceum), convulsive seizures, and mental retardation (Voigt's triad). There are primary and secondary criteria for the diagnosis of TSC. The primary criteria include adenoma sebaceum, ungual fibroma, cortical tubers, subependymal nodules, and multiple retinal astrocytomas. Among the secondary are infantile spasms, ash leaf spots (hypomelanotic lesions only seen with the Wood's lamp), cardiac rhabdomyoma, renal angiolipoma, and a first-degree relative with TSC.

Diagnosis is clinical at most ages, according to the primary and secondary criteria. Computed tomography (CT) and MRI can identify cortical tubers and subependymal giant-cell astrocytomas, among other lesions.

Treatment is nonspecific. Surgery may be indicated occasionally for tubers and astrocytomas. Antiepileptic drugs can help with infantile spasms and other seizure disorders.

A mild form of TSC can be static; patients with a full-blown syndrome have a progressive course with development of brain tumors, renal insufficiency, cardiac failures, and so forth.

Neurofibromatosis Type 1 (von Recklinghausen's Disease)

Neurofibromatosis type 1 (NF-1) is a common disorder, with a prevalence of 1 in 3,000. It is autosomal dominant (chromosome 17). The gene product is neurofibromin, a tumor suppressor gene.

Clinical manifestations include *café au lait* spots (six or more), axillary freckles, Lisch nodules (white hamartomas in the iris), multiple cutaneous tumors, multiple subcutaneous tumors (plexiform neuromas), optic glioma, spinal root tumors, neurofibromas, obstructive hydrocephalus, pheochromocytoma, and learning disabilities.

Diagnosis is based on clinical symptoms and signs, radiology, genetics, and pathologic findings. There is no specific treatment.

Neurofibromatosis Type 2 (Central Neurofibromatosis)

Neurofibromatosis type 2 (NF-2) is less common than NF-1. It is also inherited in an autosomal dominant manner (chromosome 22). The gene product is merlin.

Clinical manifestations include bilateral acoustic neuromas (neuroma in the vestibular portion of the eighth cranial nerve). The first symptom is often hearing loss due to compression of the cochlear component of the eighth cranial nerve (usually around age 20). Solitary or multicentric meningiomas are common.

Diagnosis is based on clinical symptoms and signs, radiology, genetics, and pathological findings. There is no specific treatment.

◆ KEY POINTS ◆

1. Seizures, mental retardation, and adenoma sebaceum are characteristic clinical features of TSC.

2. NF-1 is more of a "peripheral disease," whereas NF-2 is a "central" one.

3. NF-2 presents with bilateral acoustic neuromas and meningiomas.

THE HYPOTONIC INFANT

Hypotonia is a reduction in postural tone. It may be the manifestation of a central or peripheral nervous system disorder, or both. There are many causes of hypotonia in the infant.

Central hypotonia is usually related to a CNS insult (e.g., chromosomal disorder, peroxisomal disorders, metabolic defects). Central hypotonia is usually associated with developmental delay, occasional seizures, microcephaly, dysmorphic features, congenital malformations, and persistent infantile reflexes. In general, the cause of central hypotonia can be diagnosed by history and physical exam, remembering that the most striking feature is not the hypotonia but the other abnormal CNS functions.

Peripheral hypotonia can result from spinal cord problems, anterior horn cell lesions (spinal muscular atrophy), peripheral neuropathy, neuromuscular junction abnormalities, and myopathies (congenital, metabolic, etc.). The physical exam and the absence of "central" signs may help in localizing the site of pathology. Remember that infants with severe hypotonia but only marginal weakness usually do not have a disorder of the lower motor unit.

◆ KEY POINTS ◆

1. Hypotonia can be central, peripheral, or both.

2. Central hypotonia is usually associated with other signs of central nervous system dysfunction (seizures, developmental delay, etc.).

3. Infants with severe hypotonia but only marginal weakness usually do not have a disorder of the lower motor unit.

INHERITED NEURODEGENERATIVE DISEASES OF CHILDHOOD

The inherited neurodegenerative diseases are classified according to the involved cellular element: the lysosome, peroxisome, mitochondria, Golgi apparatus, and the cell membrane. Whatever the cellular and molecular mechanism responsible, it is possible to recognize common patterns of disease expression according to the age of onset, symptoms, and systems involved. The most common clinical features of neurometabolic diseases presenting in infancy and childhood are developmental delay or regression.

TABLE 25-5

Some Inherited Neurodegenerative Disorders

Disorder	Incidence and Inheritance	Metabolic Defect	Mutation	Clinical Characteristics
Lysosomal disorders				
Tay-Sachs disease (gangliosidosis)	1:4000 in Ashkenazi Jews; 1:400,000 otherwise. Autosomal recessive	Hexosaminidase A deficient and B increased (accumulates GM-2 ganglioside)	Hex A: chromosome 15; hex B: chromosome 5	Normal development for 4–6 months. Myoclonic jerks, macular cherry-red spot. Floppy baby. Hyperreflexia. Seizures, decortication, and macrocephaly. Death by age 3.
Niemann-Pick disease	1:20,000 to 40,000 in Ashkenazi Jews; autosomal recessive	Acid sphingomyelinase (accumulates sphingomyelin)	Chromosome 11	Infantile form presents with developmental regression, dementia, hypotonia, hepatomegaly, macular cherry-red spot, and death by age 2. Juvenile form presents with seizures, spasticity, vertical gaze paresis.
Gaucher's disease	1:16,000 in Ashkenazi Jews; autosomal recessive	Glucosylceramide β-glucosidase	Chromosome 1	Infantile form presents with regression, poor feeding, seizures, spasticity, macular cherry-red spot. Death by age 2. Juvenile form has dementia, seizures, splenomegaly. Adult form characterized by splenomegaly and thrombocytopenia.
Krabbe's disease (globoid cell leukodystrophy)	1:50,000 in Sweden; 1:200,000 otherwise. Autosomal recessive	Galactosylceramide β-galactosidase	Chromosome 14	Infantile Krabbe's starts between 1 and 5 years of age. Neurologic signs include irritability, rigidity, optic ataxia, gait difficulty, vision loss, cortical blindness, seizure. Peripheral neuropathy present. Progressive psychomotor deterioration. Mentation often spared. CSF protein elevated. MRI shows demyelination.
Metachromatic leukodystrophy	1:40,000; autosomal recessive	Arylsulfatase A	Chromosome 22	Produces white matter disease. Multiple phenotypes of varying age of onset and rate of progression. Onset for late infantile form is 6–24 months of age. Death in 5–6 years. Neurologic signs include gait difficulty, hypotonia, ataxia, rapid intellectual deterioration, and

				dementia. Macular cherry-red spots. Peripheral neuropathy. Hepatosplenomegaly is present as well as skeletal deformity. CSF protein elevated. Urine sulfatide test is positive. MRI shows diffuse demyelination sparing subcortical U-fibers.
Mucopolysaccharidoses (Hurler's disease)	1:150,000; autosomal recessive	α-Iduronidase	Chromosome 4	Severe dysmorphic features, skeletal deformities, and psychomotor deterioration. Appearance is normal at birth. Disease develops during first year of life. Macroglossia, glaucoma, hypertelorism present. Abnormal gait. Sensorineural deafness. Hepatosplenomegaly present as well.
Neuronal ceroid lipofuscinoses	1:13,000	Lysosomal palmitoyl protein thioesterase	Chromosome 1	Infantile form is rapidly progressive. Onset 6–20 months. Characterized by severe psychomotor deterioration, blindness with macular degeneration, microcephalia, hypotonia, ataxia, and myoclonic epilepsy. Choreoathetosis may be noted earlier.
Peroxisomal disorders				
Adrenoleukodystrophy	1:100,000; X-linked; most frequent leukodystrophy in adults and children	ATP-binding protein defect; accumulation of very long chain fatty acids (VLCFA)		Symptoms start at age 5–8 years. Infants are hypotonic, have failure to thrive, dementia, hyperreflexia, dysmorphic facies, hepatomegaly, and retinitis pigmentosa. Progressive neurologic deterioration is characterized by seizures, blindness, psychomotor retardation, and spasticity. MRI shows demyelination occipital to frontal. Spares subcortical U-fibers.
Zellweger's syndrome (cerebrohepatorenal syndrome)	1:50,000	Peroxisome membrane protein; accumulation of VLCFA		Affected newborns are poorly responsive, severely hypotonic, with arthrogryposis, dysmorphic features, cirrhosis, retinal degeneration, and cerebral malformation. Diagnosis is by accumulation of VLCFA.

Lysosomal disorders are caused by genetic defects of lysosomal enzymes and cofactors that result in the accumulation of undegraded substrates in lysosomes. They are classified according to the accumulated material: sphingolipidoses, mucopolysaccharidoses, mucolipidoses, glycogen storage disease type II, sialidoses, and neuronal ceroid lipofuscinosis. Some of the most important characteristics of these clinical entities are reviewed in Table 25–5.

Peroxisomal disorders include a heterogeneous group of syndromes characterized by abnormalities in lipid metabolism. Multiple enzyme deficiencies have been characterized. They are rare. The most important are X-linked adrenoleukodystrophy and Zellweger's syndrome (see Table 25–5). Most of the degenerative diseases of infancy and childhood are not treatable. However, attempts to reach a final diagnosis are important in order to provide parents with genetic counseling, prognosis, and further management advice.

◆ KEY POINTS ◆

1. Neurodegenerative diseases involving the white matter include metachromatic leukodystrophy, Krabbe's disease, adrenoleukodystrophy, Pelizaeus-Merzbacher disease, Canavan's disease, and Alexander's disease.

2. Peripheral nerve involvement is found in metachromatic leukodystrophy, Krabbe's disease, Canavan's disease, and adrenoleukodystrophy.

3. Congenital macular cherry-red spots (red color of the macula compared with a pale retina) are found in Tay-Sachs disease, Sandhoff disease, Niemann-Pick disease, Gaucher's disease, metachromatic leukodystrophy, and sialidoses.

Questions

1. A 78-year-old woman with dementia and rigidity is hospitalized with dehydration. During her hospitalization she becomes agitated and has prominent visual hallucinations. After a dose of haloperidol, she becomes very rigid and mute. The most likely type of dementia in this patient is:

   a. Alzheimer's disease
   b. Parkinson's disease
   c. Dementia with Lewy bodies
   d. Pick's disease

2. A 32-year-old woman presents to the emergency room complaining of blurred vision and pain in the right eye. Your evaluation shows decreased visual acuity in the right eye that does not correct with pinhole testing. There is a relative afferent pupillary defect (RAPD) on the right, and right visual field testing shows a small central scotoma. The most likely localization of the lesion is:

   a. Optic chiasm
   b. Optic nerve
   c. Optic tract
   d. Occipital cortex

3. In the same patient, ophthalmoscopic examination will likely show:

   a. Normal optic disc
   b. Swelling of the optic disc
   c. Retinal hemorrhage
   d. Drusen

4. A few months later the same patient returns to the emergency room with horizontal diplopia. Your evaluation shows normal right lateral gaze but difficulty with adduction of the right eye while looking to the left and nystagmus in the abducting left eye. The most likely cause of this clinical picture is:

   a. One-and-a-half syndrome
   b. A right internuclear ophthalmoplegia (INO)
   c. A left INO
   d. Bilateral INOs

5. In this patient, the most likely cause for all of her findings is:

   a. Stroke
   b. Multiple sclerosis
   c. Pontine hemorrhage
   d. Right frontal infarct

6. A 54-year-old woman was seen in the emergency room complaining of a severe headache. Head CT was normal, and a lumbar puncture was performed. The opening pressure was 14 cm H_2O, and CSF analysis showed the following: 150 red blood cells, xanthochromic fluid, protein 55 (slightly increased), 15 white blood cells (90% lymphocytes), and normal glucose. Which of the following statements is true?

   a. The xanthochromia may have been caused by a traumatic tap

   b. The lymphocytic pleocytosis indicates an active infectious process

   c. Viral meningitis is unlikely because of the normal CSF glucose

   d. The lymphocytic pleocytosis is likely reactive to the presence of blood within the cerebrospinal fluid

7. A 29-year-old woman is brought into the emergency room in an unresponsive state. Her temperature is 37°C, heart rate 84 per minute, respirations 10, and blood pressure 152/84. On examination, she withdraws only to noxious stimulation. Her right pupil is 10 mm and does not constrict to light. Her left pupil is 5 mm and reacts normally. Which of the following would not be appropriate in this patient's management?

   a. Raising the head of the bed

   b. Intravenous administration of mannitol

   c. Hyperventilation

   d. Lumbar puncture

   e. Neurosurgical consultation

8. A patient presents with gradually worsening weakness of the proximal arm and leg muscles symmetrically over several months. On examination, neck flexors and extensors are found to be weak also. There is no muscle pain or tenderness. What is the most likely site of dysfunction in the nervous system?

   a. Peripheral nerve

   b. Brachial plexus

   c. Spinal nerve root

   d. Internal capsule

   e. Muscle

9. An 8-year-old boy is brought to a child psychiatrist for evaluation of potential attention deficit hyperactivity disorder. His mother states that his teachers have been concerned about his attention because they frequently have to repeat instructions to him. At home his brother has noticed that he will stare for several seconds at a time, during which he does not respond to questions. An EEG demonstrates a 3-Hz spike-and-wave pattern. Which of the following is the most appropriate treatment?

   a. Methylphenidate (Ritalin)

   b. Ethosuximide (Zarontin)

   c. Clonidine (Catapres)

   d. Fluoxetine (Prozac)

   e. Carbamazepine (Tegretol)

10. Which of the following medications is least effective for preventive treatment of migraine headaches in an otherwise healthy individual?

   a. Propranolol

   b. Sumatriptan

   c. Verapamil

   d. Amitriptyline

11. A 42-year-old man is brought to the neurologist for evaluation of a few months' history of personality changes. His family indicates that over the past year he has had unusual movements of his hands and he seems to have some memory difficulties. His father died in his 50s with a similar clinical syndrome, with prominent chorea and dementia. The most likely genetic abnormality will be localized on chromosome:

   a. 19

   b. 6

   c. 4

   d. 11

12. A 55-year-old woman with a history of ovarian cancer and moderate alcohol consumption is seen in the neurology ambulatory clinic with a one-month history of progressive unsteadiness of gait and dysarthria. Examination confirms the presence

of both gait and limb ataxia as well as nystagmus. These symptoms were fairly abrupt in onset, progressed over a period of a few weeks, and now appear to have stabilized, but there has been no sign of spontaneous improvement. Which of the following statements is correct?

a. The findings of gait ataxia, dysarthria, and nystagmus indicate diffuse involvement of the cerebellum and suggest that the alcohol consumption is the likely cause

b. The constellation of symptoms and temporal evolution of her symptoms are most consistent with paraneoplastic cerebellar degeneration, a disorder associated with underlying gynecologic malignancy

c. The constellation of symptoms and temporal evolution of her symptoms are most consistent with paraneoplastic cerebellar degeneration, but ovarian cancer is an unusual cause of this syndrome

d. The symptoms and signs indicate cerebellar hemisphere dysfunction and are most suggestive of a metastasis from the underlying ovarian cancer

13. A 45-year-old man with multiple sclerosis comes to the neurology clinic complaining of urinary incontinence. He indicates that he experiences increased urgency and frequency of urination. The most likely urodynamic finding in this patient is:

a. An atonic bladder

b. A spastic bladder

c. Stress incontinence

d. None of the above

14. Which one of the following therapies can be used to treat this patient's urinary problem?

a. Tolterodine

b. Oxybutynin

c. Imipramine

d. All of the above

15. A 35-year-old man is seen in the neurology outpatient clinic with the complaint that his fingers occa-

sionally seem to "get stuck" when he is engaged in tasks like opening jars. On examination you find subtle weakness of the fingers and toes as well as percussion myotonia. You also note prominent frontal balding and suspect the diagnosis of myotonic dystrophy. Which of the following statements is false?

a. Myotonic dystrophy is the most common inherited skeletal muscle disorder that affects adults

b. It is caused by a CAG triplet expansion in the DMPK gene

c. It is a multisystem disease with manifestations including cataracts, dysphagia, frontal balding, and cardiac conduction defects

d. CK is typically normal or only mildly elevated and electromyography demonstrates myotonia

16. Which of the following is not a recognized complication of diabetes?

a. Radiculopathy

b. Cranial neuropathy

c. Myopathy

d. Peripheral neuropathy

17. A 40-year-old woman with systemic lupus erythematosus develops weakness of her right finger and wrist extensors and pain on the right dorsum of her hand several months after being diagnosed with left carpal tunnel syndrome and right sciatic neuropathy. What is the most likely diagnosis?

a. Mononeuropathy multiplex

b. Axonal polyneuropathy

c. Demyelinating polyneuropathy

d. Neuromuscular junction disease

e. Polyradiculopathy

18. A 70-year-old man develops the acute onset of an inability to speak. Examination reveals that he struggles to pronounce a complete word and cannot string words together. He is unable to repeat a sentence, but can follow simple and multistep commands. What is the most likely diagnosis?

a.   Global aphasia

b.   Conduction aphasia

c.   Broca's aphasia

d.   Wernicke's aphasia

e.   Transcortical motor aphasia

19. A 28-year-old woman is brought to the emergency room by her husband. In addition to having neck stiffness, she has had a fever for the past several days and has been somewhat confused and has not been "acting like herself." Lumbar puncture shows 9 white blood cells with a lymphocytic predominance, 32 red blood cells, protein = 63, and glucose = 65. Gram stain is negative. What is the most likely diagnosis?

a.   Bacterial meningitis

b.   Viral meningitis

c.   Fungal meningitis

d.   Meningitis from tuberculosis

20. While in the emergency room, the above patient has a generalized seizure. The onset of the seizure was not witnessed. MRI of the brain with gadolinium shows contrast enhancement of both temporal lobes. EEG shows sharp wave discharges in the temporal lobes. These new findings in conjunction with the above CSF profile are most likely to result from infection by what organism?

a.   Enterovirus or arbovirus

b.   *Streptococcus pneumoniae*

c.   *Cryptococcus neoformans*

d.   Herpes simplex virus (HSV-1)

21. Two days after coronary artery bypass surgery a 62-year-old man with hypertension complains that "there is another man's arm in bed" with him. When asked to hold up his arms, the patient raises his right arm only. When asked about his left arm, he claims it is the examiner's or another patient's. What is the most likely diagnosis?

a.   Right hemisphere stroke with neglect

b.   Left hemisphere stroke with neglect

c.   Conversion disorder

d.   Adjustment disorder

e.   Alien limb phenomenon

22. Which of the following is the initial medication used in the treatment of status epilepticus?

a.   Benzodiazepines

b.   Barbiturates

c.   Propofol

d.   Carbamazepine

e.   Lamotrigine

23. A 34-year-old woman with multiple sclerosis develops double vision upon looking to one side. Examination reveals normal eye movements except that on attempted leftward conjugate gaze, the right eye does not adduct properly and the left eye has abducting nystagmus. What is the neuroanatomic structure most likely affected?

a.   Internal capsule

b.   Oculomotor nucleus

c.   Spinal trigeminal nucleus

d.   Optic nerve

e.   Medial longitudinal fasciculus

24. Which of the following is not a treatment used in patients with multiple sclerosis?

a.   Interleukin 10 (IL-10)

b.   Interferon beta-1a

c.   Glatiramer acetate

d.   Methylprednisolone

e.   Azathioprine

25. A 75-year-old man is brought to the emergency room after having briefly lost consciousness in his bathroom. By the time he arrives in the emergency room he is feeling fine and is able to give a clear account of what happened. He recalls walking to the bathroom to urinate. Shortly thereafter he became light-headed and felt as if his vision was graying out. These symptoms lasted for about 30 seconds, and the next thing he recalls is awakening on his bathroom floor. His wife notes that he was unconscious only briefly. He is diagnosed with syncope. Which of the following descriptions pertinent to this clinical scenario is correct?

a. The symptoms of light-headedness and graying out of vision are atypical symptoms described by patients with syncope

b. He has micturition syncope, a form of neurogenic syncope that involves the reflex triggering of cardio-inhibitory and/or vasodepressor responses

c. Orthostatic hypotension is the likely explanation for his syncopal episode

d. None of the above

26. A 17-year-old girl is seen in the ambulatory neurology clinic with a six-month history of tremor and ataxia. There is no family history of neurologic disease. On examination she is noted to have subtle chorea as well as a golden brown discoloration of the cornea. Which of the following diagnoses should you suspect?

a. Sydenham's chorea

b. Wilson's disease

c. Huntington's chorea

d. Tourette's syndrome

27. Which of the following statements regarding sarcoidosis is not true?

a. Cranial neuropathy due to chronic basal meningitis is the most common manifestation of neurosarcoidosis

b. The typical pathology is that of caseating granulomata

c. When sarcoidosis affects the nervous system, it is usually in conjunction with other systemic manifestations of the disease

d. Steroids are the mainstay of therapy

28. A 64-year-old man with a history of hypertension presents to the emergency room with the sudden onset of numbness of his left leg, arm, and face. His motor examination is normal. Where is the most likely site of his lesion?

a. Right thalamus

b. Left thalamus

c. Left postcentral gyrus

d. Right precentral gyrus

29. Tearing of the middle meningeal artery will result in what type of hemorrhage?

a. Subdural hematoma

b. Epidural hematoma

c. Subarachnoid hemorrhage

d. Intracerebral hemorrhage

30. Which of the following syndromes or diseases could cause bilateral weakness and loss of pain and temperature sensation with preservation of joint position sense in both legs?

a. Amyotrophic lateral sclerosis (ALS)

b. Vitamin B_{12} deficiency

c. Brown-Séquard syndrome

d. Anterior spinal artery syndrome

31. A 2-year-old child presents with new seizures. Her mother tells you that the child is not walking yet. He has a 5-year-old brother with a seizure disorder and mental retardation. On examination, you find hypomelanotic lesions using the Wood's lamp. The most appropriate next test is:

a. Skeletal surveillance

b. Skin biopsy

c. Head CT or MRI

d. No need for further tests

32. Genetic analysis will likely show abnormalities on chromosome:

a. 19

b. 15

c. 4

d. 9

33. A 62-year-old woman with a history of small cell lung carcinoma presents to the neurology clinic complaining of bilateral lower extremity paresthesias. She has no history of diabetes or family history of polyneuropathy. She describes severe pain in the soles of her feet when standing and has difficulty walking. On examination, there is severe pain to light touch over both soles. On your sensory examination description, you will state that this patient has:

a.   Hyperesthesia

b.   Paresthesia

c.   Allodynia

d.   None of the above

34.   Treatment of this patient with gabapentin produces some improvement of her pain. Three months later, she returns to the emergency room with weakness in her lower extremities and urinary incontinence. Your examination shows a sensory level at T8. The most likely localization of the lesion is:

a.   Lumbosacral polyradiculopathy

b.   Right parietal stroke

c.   Neuromuscular junction

d.   Spinal cord

35.   A 35-year-old woman presents to the emergency room with a few days of progressive ascending muscle weakness. She had a viral infection a few weeks ago. On examination you find diffuse weakness and areflexia. The most likely finding in the spinal fluid is:

a.   High protein–high cell count

b.   High protein–low cell count

c.   Low protein–high cell count

d.   Low protein–low cell count

36.   Nerve conduction studies will likely show:

a.   Marked denervation

b.   Demyelination

c.   Axonal loss

d.   Normal

37.   You decide to treat this patient. The most appropriate therapy is:

a.   Intravenous methylprednisolone

b.   Intravenous immunoglobulins (IVIg)

c.   High doses of vitamin B_{12}

d.   Cyclophosphamide

38.   A 53-year-old woman is seen in the office complaining of dizziness. She reports that when she awoke two days ago and rolled over in bed, she suddenly developed a sensation of vertigo that was accompanied by severe nausea. These symptoms were brief and subsided over a period of about 30 seconds. Over the course of the subsequent two days she has intermittently experienced similar symptoms that have been similarly brief. She has no other symptoms and a detailed neurologic examination is entirely normal apart from the presence of torsional nystagmus elicited by the Dix-Hallpike maneuver. Which of the following statements is true?

a.   This history of the combination of vertigo, nausea, and torsional nystagmus raises concern for posterior circulation ischemia and mandates further investigation

b.   The sudden onset of vertigo, nausea, and vomiting is characteristic of vestibular neuronitis, and her symptoms should resolve within 1–2 weeks

c.   The history of brief episodes of vertigo, often precipitated by movement, is almost pathognomonic of benign positional paroxysmal vertigo (BPPV), and this diagnosis is supported by the finding of nystagmus with the Dix-Hallpike maneuver

d.   Statements (a), (b), and (c) are all false

39.   Which of the following statements concerning myasthenia gravis is false?

a.   It is an autoimmune disorder caused by antibodies that are directed against the presynaptic nicotinic acetylcholine receptor

b.   Bulbar muscle weakness is common, second only to ocular muscle weakness

c.   Acetylcholinesterase inhibitors represent symptomatic treatment, but immunosuppressive therapy is required to treat the underlying immunopathology

d.   Fatiguable muscle weakness is a characteristic symptom

40.   A patient complains of difficulty chewing. On examination he is found to have decreased strength of his muscles of mastication. Which of the following cranial nerves is responsible for this motor function?

a. Trigeminal

b. Facial

c. Oculomotor

d. Glossopharyngeal

e. Hypoglossal

41. The Glasgow Coma Scale is most commonly used in which of the following conditions?

   a. Cardiac arrest

   b. Delirium

   c. Stroke

   d. Head trauma

   e. Subarachnoid hemorrhage

42. A 68-year-old man taking warfarin falls while in the hospital, is found on the floor, and is difficult to arouse. He has a new right hemiparesis. An intracranial hemorrhage is suspected. What is the most appropriate initial radiologic study?

   a. Head CT with contrast

   b. Head CT without contrast

   c. Skull x-ray

   d. Cerebral angiography

   e. Brain perfusion scan

43. A 75-year-old man presents to your office with a one-month history of progressive pain in the left temporal area and pain in his jaw while eating. On laboratory testing, the patient is found to have an elevated erythrocyte sedimentation rate (ESR) of 94. What is the treatment of choice?

   a. Sumatriptan

   b. Carbamazepine

   c. Prednisone

   d. Surgical resection of brain tumor

44. All of the following can be used in the treatment of obstructive sleep apnea except:

   a. Continuous positive airway pressure (CPAP)

   b. Weight loss

   c. Avoidance of alcohol and sedating medication

   d. Pemoline

45. A previously healthy 21-year-old presents to the emergency room after being involved in a high speed motor vehicle accident. You note that the patient is unresponsive, makes no spontaneous movement, and has a dilated pupil on the right that is nonreactive to light. What is the best explanation for these signs?

   a. Infarction of the left occipital lobe

   b. Concussion from the motor vehicle accident

   c. Uncal herniation

   d. Cervical neck fracture

46. Which of the following brain locations is least likely to be the site of an intracerebral hemorrhage caused by hypertension?

   a. Basal ganglia

   b. Pons

   c. Frontal lobe

   d. Cerebellum

47. Narcolepsy is characterized by or can be associated with all of the following except:

   a. Obesity

   b. Cataplexy

   c. Hypnagogic hallucinations

   d. Excessive daytime sleepiness

48. A 45-year-old man with a prior history of migraine headaches with aura presents to the emergency room complaining of a progressive headache for the last month that is different from his usual migraine. There is no associated nausea or vomiting. His neurologic examination is completely normal. Your next step in management should be:

   a. Brain imaging study

   b. Abortive migraine treatment

   c. Preventive migraine treatment

   d. Reassurance and discharge home

49. Which of the following features is least likely to be associated with a pituitary adenoma?

a. Headache

b. Bitemporal hemianopia

c. Endocrine dysfunction

d. Seizures

50. Signs of upper motor neuron or corticospinal tract dysfunction include all of the following except:

a. Hypotonia

b. Increased reflexes

c. Extensor plantar response

d. Weakness

51. A 67-year-old woman presents to the emergency room with new onset of headache, nausea, vomiting, and unsteadiness of gait. Her history is significant for atrial fibrillation for which she is chronically anticoagulated with warfarin. She also has a pacemaker in place. You are concerned about the possibility of a cerebellar hemorrhage. The imaging modality of choice is:

a. A CT scan because this is the imaging modality most sensitive to the presence of acute intracranial blood

b. An MRI because the blood in the posterior fossa will not be visualized on CT

c. An MRI because CT is contraindicated by the presence of a pacemaker

d. A CT scan because it provides the best images of the contents of the posterior fossa

52. Which of the following best describes a frontal type gait disorder?

a. Stooped posture, slow, shuffling, small steps, reduced arm swing

b. Impaired gait initiation, difficulty lifting the feet off the ground, small and shuffling steps

c. A stiff leg with increased adductor tone and circumduction of the hip

d. Slow, cautious, and wide-based gait

53. A 58-year-old man is seen in the neurology ambulatory clinic with a three-month history of right-sided resting tremor. On examination, he is noted to have mild masking of facial expression and there

is diminished swing of the right arm when walking. You suspect that he may have early idiopathic Parkinson's disease. Which of the following statements concerning this disorder is true?

a. Most cases are familial with mutations in the α-synuclein or parkin genes

b. It is characterized by death of dopaminergic neurons in the substantia nigra pars reticulata

c. The four cardinal features of this disorder are tremor, rigidity, bradykinesia, and postural instability

d. Impairment of vertical gaze is a common manifestation of this disorder

54. Which of the following statements concerning Duchenne's muscular dystrophy is false?

a. The disorder is allelic with Becker's muscular dystrophy

b. Inheritance is X-linked

c. The characteristic pattern of muscle involvement includes the proximal muscles of the neck, arms, and legs

d. Serum creatine kinase is typically normal or only marginally elevated

55. Dysdiadochokinesis, or difficulty with performing rapid alternating movements, is most typically associated with dysfunction of which of the following brain structures?

a. Basal ganglia

b. Medulla

c. Cerebellum

d. Parietal lobe

e. Thalamus

56. An ischemic stroke involving the right side of the pons could lead to which of the following patterns of weakness?

a. Left face weakness and right body weakness

b. Right face weakness and left body weakness

c. Right face weakness and right body weakness

d. Left arm weakness and right leg weakness

e. Right arm weakness and left leg weakness

57. A 27-year-old woman with complex partial sei-z-ures is well controlled on carbamazepine. Which of the following is a characteristic side effect of this medication?

   a. Thrombocytopenia

   b. Agitation

   c. Diabetes insipidus

   d. Nephrolithiasis

   e. Hyponatremia

58. Subarachnoid hemorrhage is commonly caused by all of the following except:

   a. Tearing of bridging veins

   b. Trauma

   c. Aneurysm rupture

   d. Bleeding from arteriovenous malformations

59. Using brain imaging, all of the following lesions typically show ring enhancement with contrast administration except:

   a. Glioblastoma multiforme

   b. Primary central nervous system lymphoma

   c. Brain abscess

   d. Toxoplasmosis of the brain

Answers

1. c (chapter 12)

The presence of visual hallucinations is an early symptom of dementia with Lewy bodies (DLB). Other characteristics include cognitive decline, fluctuations of alertness, extrapyramidal symptoms, and an extraordinary sensitivity to neuroleptics.

2. b (chapter 4)

The decreased visual acuity that does not correct with pinhole testing, an RAPD, and a central scotoma are characteristic of optic nerve disease.

3. a or b (chapter 4)

The clinical description is consistent with an acute optic neuritis. Retinal hemorrhage does not produce an RAPD. Drusen produce so-called pseudopapilledema but do not alter visual acuity in the early stages. Optic disc swelling is a possible finding in this patient, but most optic neuritis is retrobulbar, and the disc may be normal.

4. b (chapter 4)

Lesions of the medial longitudinal fasciculus (MLF) produce an INO with ipsilateral eye adduction failure and nystagmus in the contralateral abducting eye.

5. b (chapter 4)

This is a young woman who presented with an episode of optic neuritis and later with a right INO. All the other causes are unlikely to produce optic neuritis; if a or c produce an INO, it is usually accompanied by other neurologic deficits.

6. d (chapter 2)

This woman has had a subarachnoid hemorrhage. Bleeding into the subarachnoid (CSF) space typically initiates an inflammatory response, one manifestation of which is a lymphocytic pleocytosis. Xanthochromia is the result of breakdown of blood within the subarachnoid space. Its presence in a bloody CSF sample helps to distinguish intrathecal hemorrhage from a traumatic tap. The CSF glucose is typically normal in both subarachnoid hemorrhage and viral meningitis. It is frequently low in bacterial, mycobacterial, and carcinomatous meningitis.

7. d (chapter 3)

This patient has a clinical presentation that suggests increased intracranial pressure from a right hemisphere lesion. The "blown" right pupil suggests that herniation of the right hemisphere has compressed the right oculomotor nerve. Choices a through c are all measures that acutely decrease intracranial pressure, while neurosurgery may be needed as a more definitive intervention. Performing a lumbar puncture in this situation could be dangerous and could actually precipitate worsening herniation.

---

8. e (chapter 5)

Symmetric proximal weakness usually suggests a primary muscle problem, as does weakness of neck flexors and extensors. The absence of muscle pain and tenderness does not argue against a primary muscle pathology. The other listed choices would not usually result in this pattern of weakness.

---

9. b (chapter 15)

This child likely has absence seizures, which are frequently diagnosed after a teacher or parent notices inattention, "daydreaming," or staring episodes. Absence seizures last a few seconds each, can occur many times a day, and have a classic EEG appearance. Ethosuximide and valproic acid are typical drugs of choice.

---

10. b (chapter 10)

Sumatriptan is effective for aborting migraine headaches but is not used for preventive therapy. The other medications have been shown to be effective in decreasing the severity and frequency of attacks and are used as preventive therapy in migraine headaches.

---

11. c (chapter 12)

The case represents an early onset of dementia with associated personality changes and movement disorder (chorea). This is the classic triad of Huntington's disease. Huntington's disease is linked to chromosome 4p16.3, also known as Huntington's disease gene, encoding for a protein named huntingtin. The mutation produces an unstable CAG repeat sequence with more than 40 repeats.

---

12. b (chapter 8)

Paraneoplastic cerebellar degeneration is typically a pancerebellar syndrome with clinical manifestations including ataxia, dysarthria, and nystagmus. The underlying malignancy is typically a gynecological malignancy or breast cancer. The temporal evolution is typically that of acute or subacute onset with fairly rapid progression over weeks to months, followed by stabilization. Metastatic cerebellar disease would more likely affect a cerebellar hemisphere and produce lateralized cerebellar dysfunction. Alcoholic cerebellar degeneration typically affects the vermis, and the characteristic manifestation is that of a gait ataxia.

---

13. b (chapter 9)

Multiple sclerosis characteristically produces an upper motor neuron bladder or spastic bladder with increased frequency and urgency.

---

14. d (chapter 9)

All these drugs have anticholinergic effects and can be used to treat spastic bladder.

---

15. b (chapter 24)

Although myotonic dystrophy is one of the triplet expansion diseases, it is a CTG expansion that occurs. It is the most common inherited skeletal muscle disorder that affects adults. Mild distal muscle weakness and myotonia are common skeletal muscle manifestations, and systemic features like cardiac conduction defects should be sought. CK is typically normal or only mildly elevated, and myotonia is readily demonstrable on electromyography.

---

16. c (chapter 18)

The neurologic complications of diabetes are protean. Peripheral neuropathy, autonomic neuropathy, cranial neuropathy, and radiculopathy are among the most common complications of poor glucose control. Diabetes, however, is not a cause of myopathy.

---

17. a (chapter 5)

The patient's current symptoms are suggestive of a right radial neuropathy. Multiple sequential mononeuropathies, each affecting a single peripheral nerve, are known as mononeuropathy multiplex. Pain is a typical feature. Patients with rheumatologic conditions are susceptible; vasculitis may be involved.

18.   c (chapter 11)

Broca's aphasia is characterized by effortful nonfluent speech and an inability to repeat, with relatively preserved comprehension. Transcortical motor aphasia is similar but features preserved repetition.

19.   b (chapter 21)

Along with the clinical picture, a CSF profile of lymphocytic pleocytosis, elevated protein, normal glucose with a negative Gram stain point to a viral or aseptic meningitis.

20.   d (chapter 21)

Streptococcus pneumoniae is a common cause of bacterial meningitis and *Cryptococcus neoformans* is a common cause of fungal meningitis. Enteroviruses and arboviruses are common causes of viral meningitis. However, the MRI shows contrast enhancement of the temporal lobes with red blood cells in the CSF that can indicate necrosis of the temporal lobes. The EEG confirms that the temporal lobes are not functioning normally. This pattern of injury is typical for infection with HSV-1. This diagnosis is important because mortality is high with HSV-1 meningitis. Treatment is with IV acyclovir and should be instituted promptly.

21.   a (chapter 11)

This patient exhibits a severe form of neglect, in which he does not recognize his left arm as his. Right frontal or parietal lesions are the most common etiology. In the alien limb phenomenon, patients retain awareness of the limb but feel that it is not under their control.

22.   a (chapter 15)

Benzodiazepines are the first agents used in the treatment algorithm for status epilepticus. Typically, phenytoin and then phenobarbital are used subsequently. Propofol is used if status epilepticus becomes refractory, while carbamazepine and lamotrigine are antiepileptic drugs that are not available in parenteral form.

23.   e (chapter 20)

The clinical description is of an internuclear ophthalmoplegia (INO). This is an uncommon but characteristic feature of multiple sclerosis and is due to demyelination affecting the medial longitudinal fasciculus.

24.   a (chapter 20)

Interleukin 10 is not used in the treatment of multiple sclerosis. Interferon beta-1a and glatiramer acetate are agents that reduce relapses and disability in relapsing-remitting MS, azathioprine is used in more refractory cases, and methylprednisolone is used in the acute treatment of relapses.

25.   b (chapter 7)

Micturition syncope is a form of reflex or neurogenic syncope that involves the triggering of cardio-inhibitory and/or vasodepressor responses. The symptoms of light-headedness and graying out of vision are typically reported by patients with syncope. Other symptoms they might report include a heavy feeling at the base of the neck, buckling at the knees, and tinnitus. Although orthostatic hypotension is a common cause of syncope, the occurrence of the syncopal episode after micturition rather than upon standing suggests that this is not the cause in this instance.

26.   b (chapter 12)

The corneal discoloration represents a Kayser-Fleischer ring, which is characteristic of Wilson's disease. The diagnosis should be confirmed with tests of serum copper and ceruloplasmin as well as a 24-hour urinary copper determination. Sydenham's chorea is a poststreptococcal immunologic disorder, and Huntington's disease is a neurodegenerative disorder characterized by chorea and dementia. Kayser-Fleischer rings are not present in either of these latter two conditions. Tourette's syndrome is a genetic disorder characterized by motor and vocal tics. Chorea is not a feature of this syndrome.

---

27. b (chapter 18)

The characteristic pathology is that of noncaseating granulomata. Neurosarcoidosis most commonly affects the nervous system as part of a more systemic disease. Cranial neuropathy due to chronic basal meningitis is the most common manifestation of the disease, with the facial nerve most often affected. Other manifestations include meningoencephalitis, seizures, myelopathy, and peripheral neuropathy.

---

28. a (chapter 14)

Because of the sudden onset of symptoms along with the patient's stroke risk factors, he most likely has had a pure sensory stroke. The most likely lesion is in the contralateral thalamus because the sensory pathways cross prior to synapsing in the thalamus. The left postcentral gyrus is on the wrong side to explain the patient's deficit. Also, it is unusual to have sensory loss of the face, arm, and leg equally from a stroke affecting the postcentral gyrus. This is because the middle cerebral artery provides blood to the face and arm regions of the cortex, while the anterior cerebral artery supplies blood to the leg region. The precentral gyrus is predominantly involved in motor pathways and not the sensory system.

---

29. b (chapter 17)

The middle meningeal artery travels between the skull and the dura. When this vessel is damaged (typically due to trauma resulting in a skull fracture that lacerates the middle meningeal artery) blood accumulates in the epidural space. Diagnosis and treatment is an emergency because the blood will continue to collect and may cause eventual brain herniation if untreated.

---

30. d (chapter 22)

ALS is a motor neuron disease with involvement of the lower motor neurons and corticospinal tracts. Weakness, muscle atrophy, and muscle fasciculations are prominent features. Sensory findings are not typical of ALS. Vitamin B_{12} deficiency classically results in degeneration of the dorsal columns and corticospinal tracts. Therefore, joint position sense loss and weakness are typical features, whereas pain and temperature are spared. Brown-Séquard syndrome results from hemisection of the spinal cord. The classic features are ipsilateral weakness and loss of joint position sense with contralateral loss of pain and temperature sensation below the lesion. Anterior spinal artery syndrome usually results from infarction of the anterior spinal artery, causing ischemia to the anterior two-thirds of the spinal cord. Therefore, dorsal columns are spared but weakness and loss of pain and temperature result because of involvement of the ventral horns and spinothalamic tracts.

---

31. c (chapter 25)

This patient meets diagnostic criteria for tuberous sclerosis complex (TSC). A head CT or MRI may identify cortical tubers, subependymal giant-cell astrocytomas, or other lesions. The other tests do not help in the evaluation of TSC.

---

32. d (chapter 25)

TSC is an autosomal dominant disease affecting chromosome 9 for TSC 1 and chromosome 16 for TSC 2. Hamartin is the gene product for TSC1, and tuberin is the gene product for TSC2. Both are considered tumor suppression genes.

---

33. c (chapter 6)

Allodynia indicates pain provoked by normally innocuous stimuli; hyperesthesia indicates increased sensitivity to sensory stimuli, and paresthesias refer to abnormal spontaneous sensations.

---

34. d (chapter 6)

The hallmark of a spinal cord lesion is a sensory level. Lumbosacral polyradiculopathy would produce a root pattern of sensory loss. Neuromuscular junction problems are not associated with sensory abnormalities. A right parietal stroke will produce a left hemisensory loss involving face, arm, and leg.

35. b (chapter 23)

The albuminocytologic dissociation means high protein with almost no cells in the CSF. It is characteristic of Guillain-Barré syndrome.

36. b or d (chapter 23)

Guillain-Barré syndrome is also known as acute inflammatory demyelinating polyradiculoneuropathy (AIDP), and the hallmark is peripheral nerve demyelination. Some demyelination may be evident within a few days on nerve conduction studies, but findings may be modest in the first week.

37. b (chapter 23)

IVIg and plasmapheresis are both appropriate treatments for AIDP. The use of steroids has not been proven to be beneficial.

38. c (chapter 7)

Patients with BPPV report episodes of vertigo that are precipitated by changes in position like turning over in bed or looking upwards. The attacks are brief, usually lasting seconds to minutes. Severe nausea and vomiting may accompany these attacks. While it is true that the onset of symptoms in vestibular neuronitis is typically abrupt, the time course is usually more prolonged with symptoms lasting around 24 hours and then resolving gradually. Isolated vertigo (even with nausea and vomiting) in the absence of other evidence of brainstem dysfunction, is rarely caused by brainstem ischemia.

39. a (chapter 24)

Myasthenia gravis is an autoimmune disorder, but the antibodies are directed against the postsynaptic nicotinic acetylcholine receptor. It should not be confused with the Lambert-Eaton myasthenic syndrome (LEMS) in

which antibodies are directed against the presynaptic voltage-gated calcium channel.

40. a (chapter 1)

The trigeminal nerve is responsible for the muscles of mastication. The facial nerve innervates the muscles of facial expression, the oculomotor nerve subserves eye movements, the glossopharyngeal nerve innervates some pharyngeal muscles, and the hypoglossal nerve moves the tongue.

41. d (chapter 3)

The Glasgow Coma Scale, which is used to provide a composite assessment of unresponsive patients based on their eye movements, motor function, and language ability, is typically used for patients after head trauma. It has prognostic value for head injury patients and is easy to use by nonphysicians.

42. b (chapter 3)

A noncontrast head CT is the imaging study of choice in suspected intracranial hemorrhage. This allows for the easiest delineation of acute blood, which should appear hyperdense (bright) on this study.

43. c (chapter 10)

The patient's clinical presentation is typical for temporal arteritis: age over 50, pain over the temporal arteries, jaw claudication, and an elevated ESR. Definitive diagnosis is made by temporal artery biopsy. Treatment with prednisone for several months must be initiated early, because involvement of the ophthalmic artery can lead to blindness if diagnosis and treatment are delayed.

44. d (chapter 13)

Pemoline, a nonamphetamine stimulant, is used for the treatment of narcolepsy. Obstructive sleep apnea is characterized by repetitive episodes of upper airway obstruction during sleep. CPAP helps maintain airway patency. Alcohol and sedating drugs can decrease upper airway tone, resulting in worsening symptoms. Lastly, obesity is a risk factor for obstructive sleep apnea, so weight loss may be beneficial in obese patients.

---

45.   c (chapter 17)

Uncal herniation results from mass lesions of the middle cranial fossa. This patient most likely has a hemorrhage in the middle cranial fossa from head trauma. If large enough, the mass lesion causes displacement of the medial portion of the temporal lobe (uncus) downward over the tentorium cerebelli. This typically results in compression of the brainstem and entrapment of the third cranial nerve. This compression can cause coma due to disruption of the ascending arousal system from the brainstem. It causes an ipsilateral dilated pupil due to compression of the parasympathetic nerve fibers (traveling with the third cranial nerve) that normally cause pupillary constriction.

---

46.   c (chapter 14)

Intracerebral hemorrhages caused by hypertension are most often found in the basal ganglia, thalamus, pons, and cerebellum in order of decreasing frequency. Hemorrhage into a lobe of the brain (lobar hemorrhage) is usually caused by a bleeding diathesis, trauma, or underlying lesion such as brain tumor or amyloid angiopathy.

---

47.   a (chapter 13)

Obesity can be associated with obstructive sleep apnea. Narcolepsy is characterized by excessive daytime sleepiness and can be associated with cataplexy and other REM sleep phenomena such as hypnagogic hallucinations or sleep paralysis.

---

48.   a (chapter 19)

A headache that is either different from the normal pattern or progressive deserves to be investigated further with a brain imaging study. Slowly progressive brain tumors can be associated with a normal neurologic exam or minor abnormalities. Nausea and vomiting need not be present, especially in the early stages of a tumor.

---

49.   d (chapter 19)

Seizures are not usually a feature of pituitary adenoma. Headache, endocrine dysfunction, and bitemporal hemianopia (visual field deficit in bilateral temporal visual fields) are typically seen to varying degrees.

---

50.   a (chapter 22)

Signs of upper motor neuron or corticospinal tract dysfunction include hypertonia, spasticity, increased reflexes, and an extensor plantar response (Babinski sign). Signs of lower motor neuron dysfunction include hypotonia, decreased or absent reflexes, and a flexor plantar response (down-going toe). Weakness is present with either upper or lower motor neuron dysfunction.

---

51.   a (chapter 2)

CT is the imaging modality of choice for demonstrating acute intracranial bleeding. While it is true that MRI provides better visualization of the contents of the posterior fossa, a cerebellar hemorrhage will be visible on CT. Patients with pacemakers and other implanted metal objects cannot undergo MRI.

---

52.   b (chapter 8)

The typical frontal gait is characterized by impaired initiation, difficulty lifting the feet off the ground, and small, shuffling steps. a is a description of a parkinsonian gait, c describes a hemiplegic gait and d is that of an ataxic gait.

---

53.   c (chapter 12)

Pathologically, Parkinson's disease is characterized by progressive death of dopaminergic neurons of the substantia nigra pars compacta. Most cases of Parkinson's disease are sporadic, but there are reports of familial cases in which mutations in the parkin and α-synuclein genes have been described. Impairment of vertical gaze is a common feature of progressive supranuclear palsy (PSP), a neurodegenerative disorder that is also characterized by parkinsonian features.

54. d (chapter 24)

Serum kinase is typically markedly elevated in Duchenne's muscular dystrophy. Duchenne's muscular dystrophy and Becker's muscle dystrophy both result from mutations in the *dystrophin* gene. The disorder is inherited in an X-linked manner most often affecting young boys. Proximal muscle weakness is characteristic with relative sparing of ocular and bulbar muscles.

55. c (chapter 1)

The cerebellum is the primary brain structure involved in coordination, although other components of the motor pathways are involved as well. Testing for rapid alternating movements is part of the coordination exam. The other choices listed have little or no primary role in coordination.

56. b (chapter 5)

"Crossed signs" can occur with unilateral lesions in the pons, if descending motor fibers heading for the ipsilateral facial nucleus are affected with the descending fibers heading for the contralateral spinal cord. With right pontine lesions, the right face and left body could be weak.

57. e (chapter 15)

Characteristic side effects of carbamazepine include hyponatremia, agranulocytosis, and the risk for Stevens-Johnson syndrome. Except for the hyponatremia, these side effects are rare.

58. a (chapter 14)

Tearing of bridging veins is the underlying mechanism for a subdural hematoma. Trauma is the most common cause for subarachnoid hemorrhage. Because arteries are located in the subarachnoid space, ruptured aneurysms and hemorrhage from arteriovenous malformations result in subarachnoid hemorrhage.

59. b (chapter 19)

Primary central nervous system lymphoma usually shows diffuse, homogeneous enhancement. The other lesions all show ring enhancement after contrast administration.

Index